Organizational Transformation in Health Care

Heather A. Andrews
Lynn M. Cook
Janet M. Davidson
Donald P. Schurman
Eric W. Taylor
Ronald H. Wensel

Foreword by Don Berwick
Chapter Four contributed by Jim Selman

Organizational Transformation in Health Care

A Work in Progress

Jossey-Bass Publishers • San Francisco

Substantial discounts on bulk quantities of Jossey-Bass books are available to corporations, professional associations, and other organizations. For details and discount information, contact the special sales department at Jossey-Bass Inc., Publishers.
(415) 433-1740; Fax (415) 433-0499.

Manufactured in the United States of America. Nearly all Jossey-Bass books and jackets are printed on recycled paper that contains at least 50 percent recycled waste, including 10 percent post-consumer waste. Many of our materials are also printed with either soy- or vegetable-based ink; during the printing process these inks emit fewer volatile organic compounds (VOCs) than petroleum-based inks. VOCs contribute to the formation of smog.

Library of Congress Cataloging-in-Publication Data

Organizational transformation in health care : a work in progress /
    Heather A. Andrews . . . [et al.].—1st ed.
        p.   cm.—(A joint publication in the Jossey-Bass health series
    and the Jossey-Bass management series)
    Includes bibliographical references and index.
    ISBN 0-7879-0037-0
    1. Health services administration—Canada. 2. Total quality
management. I. Andrews, Heather A. II. Series: Jossey-Bass health series.
III. Series: Jossey-Bass management series.
    [DNLM: 1. Delivery of Health Care—organization & administration—Canada.
2. Delivery of Health Care—trends—Canada. 3. Total quality management.
4. Organizational Innovation. 5. Quality of Health Care—organization &
administration—Canada. W 84 DC2)6 1994]
RA971.0686 1994
362.1'0971—dc20
DNLM/DLC
for Library of Congress   94-25556
                                                 CIP

FIRST EDITION
HB Printing   10 9 8 7 6 5 4 3 2 1   Code 94119

A joint publication in the Jossey-Bass Health Series
and the Jossey-Bass Management Series

Contents

Tables, Figures, and Exhibits

Foreword

Academic medical centers are the secular cathedrals of our time. Nowhere is this more evident than in the soaring spaces of the medical complex at the University of Alberta Hospital* in Edmonton. Tiers of balconies overlook tiled prairies of arcades and atria, the whole glowing under enormous skylights. It is as if someone let the plains inside, but without the sometimes bitter cold and wind of this part of the world. It is a safe place to learn and heal, but also an ambitious one.

With this privileged status come serious responsibilities. Centers like this are supposed to be beacons for all who are committed to improving the state of health of individuals and their communities. The academic medical center ensures the development of future professions, increases the store of knowledge that provides the basis for this work, and offers a last, best place of caring for those whose illnesses require the most advanced medical technologies. They are supposed to carve the future.

On the whole, academic centers have borne these responsibilities admirably. Diagnostic and imaging sciences have made the exploration of disease safer and more complete, and treatment technologies now save the lives of tiny newborns, trauma victims,

*Although the official title for the hospital is plural—the University of Alberta Hospitals—for ease of grammar, the organization will be referred to in the singular throughout the text.

cancer patients, and many others who only a few decades ago were doomed. University centers have contributed as well to less glamorous but even more powerful innovations in community medicine and public health. It was academic investigators who developed treatment breakthroughs for infant oral rehydration, contraception, and immunization, and public health researchers continue to advance understanding of the behavioral and sociological components of community development and primary care.

But this rich history of contribution to our knowledge and care has not been enough to keep out the prairie winds of change that now blow hard against the health care systems of the United States and Canada. Progress has been great in medicine, but something has gone wrong—so wrong that governments and public payers are now insistent that major systemic changes must be made. The most important issue, of course, is cost. Health care in the United States has reached almost 15 percent of the GNP, and, although Canada is still considerably lower, the rate of growth in health care costs has caused almost equal alarm there.

Strong research suggests that the key cost driver is the supply of services. Unlike other industries, in which costs tend to fall as supply increases, the dynamics of health care produce an upward cost spiral as more doctors, more hospitals, and more technologies become available. Supply one Magnetic Resonance Imager, and community use will be x. Supply two, and the use will rise to $2x$. Three scanners make $3x$, and so on, without much apparent limit. If we double the number of hospital beds per capita, we harvest nearly double the hospital bed-days of care, other factors being equal.

The simple, favorable explanation—that unmet needs are satisfied by increasing the supply of services—has not withstood investigation. There is little evidence that, among Western nations, those with high use and high cost of care harvest higher health status as a result. In fact, there is little relationship among the Western democracies between the health status of a population and the expenditure per capita for health care in that population. The

United States stands by far first in care costs per capita, but twenty-first among nations in infant mortality.

Without evidence of benefit from the costs, the payers in the countries with the two most costly health care systems in the world—the United States and Canada—would be fools not to raise questions. They are not fools. They know full well that unneeded expenditures for health care are expenditures denied to other useful social sectors—education, housing, and environment, for example—or at the very least, crassly, profits denied to stockholders.

As helpful as they have been in advancing medical science and practice, academic medical centers have, overall, not yet engaged effectively the scientific and educational challenges of this other modern concern: healing they system of care in which they themselves exist. Instead, committed to their traditions, proud of their pasts, and fully devoted to their current pursuits of knowledge, education and high-tech patient care, academic medical centers have, on the whole, joined their partners in the system of care—community-based institutions, professional societies, and medical trade associations—in resisting change. They have clung tightly to their current, familiar roles in the current, familiar system, instead of taking on wholeheartedly the task of redesigning the system itself. Most academic medical centers have some strategic plan for reacting to environmental pressures, but few, if any, have yet forged and acted on a guiding vision of the new system of care that they intend to help create and lead.

Slowly, painfully, but clearly, the University of Alberta Hospital in Edmonton is emerging as one among the rare exceptions. This book bears witness not to a struggle for self-preservation, but rather to the embracing of change in service to society. Here a group of capable and insightful managers, led by a man of true vision, Don Schurman, reveal their own hard work toward reinventing their cathedral.

We should take note not only of their intent but also of their style. As befits a center of academic leadership, these efforts are fully informed by theory, by study, and by invention. Don Schurman and his colleagues have spared no pains in searching the world for experts and knowledge that can help them improve. Like the best of scientists, they have reviewed the literature in many nooks and crannies for concepts that might help them. As a result, like the best of scientists, they have created something new: their own disciplined but innovative assembly of theories and approaches that best fit their own background and circumstances, and on the basis of which they are willing to act, refining their approach to cycles of learning.

We can call what they are doing "TQM" if we like, or "CQI," or whatever seems to fit. But no matter what the label, the important conclusion is that the University of Alberta Hospital is on exactly the journey of discovery and invention that it has a duty to pursue. Unlike too many of its sister academic centers, it has decided to invent a future that is fundamentally different from its past.

Don Schurman, though an optimist, is the first to admit how tough the struggle for change is. The environment, cutting budgets and demanding change now, is extremely stressful, and in less capable hands it could irretrievably injure morale. In addition, the lag is evident between the hospital's willingness to change and the equivalent force for change among the teachers and researchers who are equally party to the future of the academic center. The severe environment has knocked first on the hospital's door, and perhaps that is why the leaders of the hospital have been slightly ahead of others in most academic centers in recognizing that the past will be a poor blueprint for the future.

The change has begun. For academic medical centers, including this one, becoming the beacons they ought to be will require that the managerial changes so thoughtfully described in this book be reflected, as well, in their teaching and research missions. Students of medicine, nursing, health administration, and allied disciplines need carefully crafted instruction in the new skills of quality management: systems thinking, group process, teamwork, statistical thinking, conflict resolution, outcomes measurement, and others. For each of these "quality sciences" there is an important and, so far, unmet research challenge: to advance the state of these arts, and to assure that these methods, derived as they have been from non-medical settings, are successfully adapted to the world of medicine and public health. For the most part, these tasks—to train our professionals to be citizens of systems improvement, and to advance the improvement of sciences themselves—are as appropriate to the academic medical center as are the more traditional endeavors to understand and to heal disease.

Few academic medical centers are today positioned better than the University of Alberta Hospital to accomplish this transition to academic leadership of a new system of care. This book documents a great beginning. By fully engaging all the forces that make an academic center special—teaching, research, and the advancement of new approaches to practice—the University of Alberta Hospital can be the leader among its breed, and continue to inspire the spirit of progress embodied in its soaring open spaces.

Boston, Massachusetts   DON BERWICK
August 1994

Preface

Organizational Transformation in Health Care: A Work in Progress is about an organization being re-created, a journey still in progress, an educational experience under way. It is the account—as it is happening—by members of the senior executive team of a major Canadian teaching hospital of their experiences with organizational transformation, total quality management, and reengineering.

Each of the authors has had a unique and valuable opportunity to be part of an executive team responsible for guiding an institution through an era of political and social change, financial constraint and upheaval, reform in the public sector, and refocusing of the locus of organizational control. Through individual responsibilities for organizational change, collective commitments within the organization, and experiences and learning as the change was (and is) occurring, significant understanding and insight into large-scale change have been gained.

The intent of this book is to share the authors' understanding, experiences, and insights with others. Organizational transformation is comparable to turning a huge ocean liner: the reform in the organization has only begun and the course is not yet certain. In fact, in the 1990s—the era of change, as it has been described—the notion of stability and a predictable course is a thing of the past. Organizations are learning to function in an environment of continual change; the objective is to create the change rather than continually be battered by it. Through the management of change, a preferred future can be created.

The philosophy that has been the cornerstone of the transformational activities within the University of Alberta Hospital was initially understood as total quality management. With a unique approach to the implementation of total quality, the authors, as the organization's leaders, have accessed and evaluated many approaches to total quality management, continuous improvement, organizational transformation, and reengineering, choosing particular aspects of each to complement the organizational needs and requirements at the time.

This book urges change agents in health care and other organizations to consider total quality management through continuous improvement and reengineering as a viable philosophical approach to the challenges facing any business. The principles underlying the philosophy promote preferred change leading to unsurpassed performance.

Who Should Read This Book?

This book is for both students and practitioners in health care and other organizations who are experiencing change, responding to change, or attempting to transform their organizations for viability and survival today and into the future. It will also be of interest to students of organization theory, change theory, and organizational behavior. Those studying administration within the health or public service sectors will benefit from an understanding of one organization's experience. Those with a curiosity about total quality management as an instrument to effect chance in an organization will benefit as well.

Overview of the Contents

Organizational Transformation in Health Care is divided into three parts. Part One introduces the Canadian health care system and the foundation on which the change initiatives are built. The essence of the application of the principles of total quality management as adopted within the organization is presented in Part Two. Each chapter focuses on one of the key principles, illustrates the manner in which the concept was applied, and describes the impact that it had in practice. One significant aspect of this presentation is the lessons that were learned from the experiences. Part Three provides a "look back" and a "look forward." Looking back, the executive team reflects on "what it's *really* like." All specific initiatives set aside, how is the organization doing with respect to the principles? Looking forward, an attempt is made to speculate on what the tumultuous future will present in terms of challenges and opportunities for health care and for organizations.

Chapter One introduces the reader to Canada and the Canadian health care system. A brief historical perspective is provided, as well as insight into the challenges being faced in the 1990s. The University of Alberta Hospital is introduced, as is the context within which it exists. Chapter Two introduces the Organization Capability Development Framework. This framework, highly valued as an anchor and an integrating mechanism in the change initiatives, has contributed significantly to the alignment and understanding of the complete picture associated with organizational transformation. In Chapter Three the framework is applied within the University of Alberta Hospital. This description provides insight into the specific aspects of the context, infrastructure, and member capability within the organization. In addition, the principles of total quality management as adopted by the organization are introduced. These form the structure for Part Two of the book.

Each chapter in Part Two is dedicated to illustrating and exploring one of the principles of total quality management as defined within the University of Alberta Hospital. Chapter Four addresses the principle of *effective relationships*. Of the learning that has occurred within the organization, a rethinking of the fundamentals associated with interrelationships and coordination of action to achieve results has been invaluable. In Chapter Five, *empowerment and decentralization* are addressed through a "shared governance" initiative developed within the Nursing Division but ultimately affecting the entire organization. The notion of *accountability* is dealt with in Chapter Six, the content of which relates to organizational structure and its implications for financial management. Chapter Seven illustrates *measurable, observable results* associated with the assessment of variability in clinical practice. This chapter is of particular interest to physicians and other health care professionals. In Chapter Eight, the principle of *process management* is explored. The specific focus is the alignment of the systems associated with performance management within the total quality context of the organization. Chapter Nine describes a project "in progress." The hospital, at the time of publication, had embarked on a reengineering initiative called the "Patient Care Design Project." The chapter provides an understanding of the initial concepts and early work. This presentation illustrates the principle of *customer satisfaction*. The final chapter in Part Two focuses on the principle of *collaboration* and explores the importance of effective working relationships with partners, including unions and other health care organizations.

Part Three seeks (1) to provide the reader with a deeper understanding of the realities of organizational transformation as they are played out in day-to-day life—a look back at the experience from the executive perspective—as well as (2) to speculate about the future of organizations, health care, and the public sector.

These twelve chapters represent the commitment to "communicate with the field" the important understandings and experiences associated with transformation of an organization based on an understanding of total quality management, continuous improvement, and reengineering. These are the perspectives of the executive team during the initial years of the transformation. The learning is still occurring, as are the changes.

Acknowledgments

There are many people we would like to thank for their role in this project. The positive support and tireless efforts of Leigh Mullaly,

Loretta Thiering, and Sharon VanDoninck in dealing with draft manuscripts is greatly appreciated. Thanks is extended to the editorial staff at Jossey-Bass for their confidence, advice, flexibility, and patience in the development of this book.

Appreciation is extended to Dr. Don Berwick for his encouragement and facilitation surrounding the project and to Jim Selman (the primary author of Chapter Four) for the challenge, learning, and development he has brought to the executive team as its primary coach.

There are many acknowledgments associated more with the implementation of total quality management in general than with this book in particular. First, to the board of the University of Alberta Hospital for their untiring support of and unwavering belief in the chosen direction of organizational change—thank you. Second, to the staff and physicians associated with the organization that understood, aligned with, and fully invested in the new direction being set for the organization—your knowledge, skills, and commitment will have a lasting impact on this organization and on the future of health care.

Last, the authors would like to acknowledge one another. It has been a great privilege to work as part of a team of people with complementary skills, personalities, and capabilities. The mutual support and encouragement, both in this book project and on an ongoing basis, have made this aspect of each of our careers valuable, memorable, and rewarding.

Edmonton, Alberta
August 1994

HEATHER A. ANDREWS
LYNN M. COOK
JANET M. DAVIDSON
DONALD P. SCHURMAN
ERIC W. TAYLOR
RONALD H. WENSEL

The Authors

Heather A. Andrews is Vice President (Patient Services) at the University of Alberta Hospital, Edmonton. She earned a nursing diploma (1968) from the hospital and a bachelor's degree in nursing (1976), a master's degree in health services administration (1978), and a doctoral degree in philosophy (Educational Administration) (1987) from the University of Alberta, Edmonton.

Andrews has coauthored two nursing texts with prominent American nursing theorist Sister Callista Roy and has published articles relating to shared governance in nursing and collaboration in organizations. She has been involved in the organizational transformation efforts at the University of Alberta Hospital for the past four years, initially as Vice President (Nursing) and now in her current position.

Lynn M. Cook is Vice President (Corporate Development) at the University of Alberta Hospital. She earned a bachelor's degree in home economics (1970) and a master's degree in business administration (1983) from the University of Alberta, Edmonton. She is a certified health executive with the Canadian College of Health Service Executives.

Cook has held numerous management positions in the private sector, in government, and in health care organizations. She is a member of the Council on the Management of Total Quality, Conference Board of Canada. Cook contributed to the corporate change initiative at the University of Alberta Hospital in the executive positions of Vice President (Support Services) and Vice President (Operations) before assuming her current portfolio.

Janet M. Davidson is Vice President (Patient Services) at the University of Alberta Hospital. She earned a nursing diploma (1969) from the Toronto East General Hospital, a bachelor's degree in nursing (1971) from the University of Windsor in Windsor, Ontario, and a master's degree in health services administration (1984) from the University of Alberta, Edmonton. She is currently a part-time doctoral student in medical sociology at the University of Alberta, Edmonton.

Davidson has over twenty years experience in health care management in the volunteer, government, and hospital sectors. She has been involved in the organization transformation efforts at the University of Alberta Hospital for the past six years, initially as director of planning and now in her present position. She is a member of the Canadian College of Health Service Executives. Additionally, she serves in a voluntary capacity on the national board of the Canadian Red Cross Society, where she currently holds the position of vice president—the first woman to be elected to this position.

Donald P. Schurman is president and chief executive officer at the University of Alberta Hospital, a position he has held since 1987. He earned a bachelor's degree in commerce (1969) from the University of Saskatchewan, Saskatoon, and a master's degree in health services administration (1979) from the University of Alberta, Edmonton.

Schurman is one of the prime proponents of the transformation of the Canadian health care system through the utilization of total quality management tools and techniques. His strategy has been to utilize the University of Alberta Hospital as a demonstration model for others in the health care system. He has written articles on the application of quality principles to health care and spoken widely throughout Canada.

Schurman is a past member of the board of the Canadian Council on Health Facility Accreditation and currently serves on the boards of the Ottawa-based National Quality Institute and the Health Care Forum in San Francisco. He also serves as chair of the Canadian Quality Healthcare Network.

Eric W. Taylor is Vice President (Corporate Support) at the University of Alberta Hospital. He earned a business diploma (1971) from the Northern Alberta Institute of Technology and received his designation as a certified general accountant (1974). He received a bachelor's degree in administration (1987) from Athabasca University, Athabasca, Alberta, and a master's degree in business administration (1990) from the University of Alberta, Edmonton.

Taylor has extensive experience in health care administration and finance and continues to be involved in teaching activities, most recently in a course in total quality management in the MBA program at the University of Alberta. He has been involved in the organizational transformation at the University of Alberta Hospital for the past four years, initially as Vice President (Finance) and now in his current position.

Ronald H. Wensel is Vice President (Patient Services) at the University of Alberta Hospital. He earned a medical degree from the University of Alberta, Edmonton (1956) and later became a fellow of the Royal College of Physicians and Surgeons of Canada (1961). He also held a National Institute of Health research fellowship at the University of Washington (1962–1963) specializing in gastroenterology.

Wensel was director of the Division of Gastroenterology (1969–1980) and president of the medical staff (1988–1990) at the University of Alberta Hospital and is the current chair of the Quality of Care Committee of the Canadian Medical Association and

president of the Association of Medical Directors of Canadian
Teaching Hospitals. He has been involved in the change process
and clinical quality improvement at the University of Alberta
Hospital for the past four years, initially as Vice President (Medical
Affairs) and now in his current position, in which he has responsi-
bility for surgical, obstetrical, and anesthetic services in the hospital.

Contributing Author

James C. Selman is chief executive officer and president of Para-
Comm Partners International, a consulting and educational firm
specializing in organizational transformation, with offices in Calgary,
Los Angeles, and San Francisco. Selman graduated with degrees in
social psychology and philosophy from the University of Oklahoma,
and has done graduate work at the University of Florida. He is a
certified management consultant and has published numerous articles on management and change, including "Coaching and the Art
of Management" (*Organizational Dynamics*, 1989) coauthored with
Dr. Roger Evered.

Since 1980, Selman has studied with Dr. Fernando Flores and
has been a primary proponent of his theories and methods, which
are based in ontological, linguistic distinctions. Selman's practice
as a consultant and coach to senior management has been widely
acknowledged as an important element in the design and effective
implementation of total quality initiatives, particularly in the service sector. He has worked with the management of the University
of Alberta Hospital since 1990.

Organizational Transformation in Health Care

Part One

Introduction

As in other industrialized countries, the 1990s will become known as an era of change and transition in Canada. One sector of the Canadian economic scene that will undergo extensive reform is the national health care system. This book is about that change: about ensuring that the quality of the system is maintained and even enhanced in the face of shrinking resources and downsizing.

To illustrate the transition, Part One explores the experience of the University of Alberta Hospital in Edmonton, which has adopted total quality management as its approach to sustaining and enhancing health care services while responding to an economic climate of constraint and reduction. This approach and the related conceptualization and principles that guide action within the organization helped the hospital develop a responsive learning culture that continues to equip individuals and groups to be creative and innovative in planning for the future while responding to the demands of the present.

Chapter One introduces the reader first to the Canadian health care system, through a brief overview of the country and its distinctive features, and then to the University of Alberta Hospital

1

and its role in the system. Chapter Two explores organizational transformation and its significance for the future. The chapter examines an organization capability framework that has proven beneficial in guiding the management of the University of Alberta Hospital as the reform in health care has affected its organization and its programs. In Chapter Three, that framework is described in terms specific to the organization. The seven key principles associated with the hospital's implementation of total quality management (TQM) are identified and briefly described. These principles form the structure for Part Two where specific initiatives are used to illustrate each principle's impact within the organization.

Chapter One

The Canadian Health Care System: An Overview

Janet M. Davidson

Canada is the largest country in the Western Hemisphere (Hoffman, 1993). Its borders stretch from the Pacific to the Atlantic and from the North Pole to the United States—an area of 3,849,000 square miles. The country is noted for its geographic diversity ranging from the rugged seacoasts of the Atlantic and the Pacific, to the spectacular beauty of the Rocky Mountains, the vast flatness of the prairies, the desolation of the Arctic islands and hinterlands, and the lush, arable valleys of the Great Lakes region. Although the climate is generally considered temperate, at its extreme it ranges from the frigid zones of the high Arctic in the winter to the blistering, humid heat of central Canada in the summer.

Canada is divided into ten provinces and two territories. The population in 1991 was 26,835,500, with 77 percent residing in urban areas. The largest city, Toronto, had a population of 3,751,000 at that time, a sharp contrast to sparsely populated, isolated settlements in the far north and throughout the territories. Canada's major industries are associated with minerals, crude oil, arable land, livestock, fishing, electrical production, and crude steel production. In 1990, the gross domestic product (GDP) was reported at $516 billion, with a per capita GDP of $19,500.*

Politically, Canada is a confederation with parliamentary democracy. Formerly a colony of the British Empire, about one-

---

*All references to dollar amounts throughout this book are in Canadian dollars.

quarter of the population is of British descent. Officially bilingual (French and English), Canada prides itself on its multiculturalism and ethnic diversity. Native Indian and Inuit peoples reside in reserved lands throughout the provinces and in the Northwest and Yukon Territories.

Health care in Canada is a public sector, not-for-profit responsibility. Life expectancy at birth in 1991 was seventy-three years for males and eighty years for females. Infant mortality per 1,000 live births was 7.3. Currently there is one hospital bed for each 148 persons and one physician for every 449 persons. For the past thirty years, Canada has enjoyed one of the world's highest standards of living while creating and maintaining a socially progressive environment. The literacy rate is reported to be 99 percent.

In common with most other first world countries, Canada faces increasing economic difficulties in a rapidly changing and competitive world. Productivity is the foundation of a country's standard of living; to achieve sustained productivity growth, an economy must continually and effectively respond to environmental change. In recent years, however, the Canadian economy has shown little evidence of renewal, making real productivity growth increasingly difficult to achieve and, perhaps more importantly, to sustain (Porter, 1991). Such growth is essential if there is to be continued support of the health care system as it is presently known.

The Canadian Health Care System

Since its inception in the 1960s, the publicly financed hospital and physician services system known as Medicare, has become a defining component of the Canadian national identity. Canadians highly value their universal health care system and are determined to sustain it in as close to its present form as possible, despite considerable economic pressure for change.

The Canadian health care system represents a partnership among individual Canadians; their provincial and federal governments; and the professional groups, institutions, and organizations involved in the provision of care. Credit for the birth of the system is generally given to the province of Saskatchewan, which first introduced broad-based hospital services insurance in the mid-1950s, followed by insured physician services in the early 1960s. Both of these social measures were subsequently championed by the federal government, which used its broad spending power to assist with the funding of a national program.

The move to publicly funded physician services was not without tumult. In 1962, the province of Saskatchewan experienced a bitter strike by physicians in protest against the launching of the provincial medical care insurance program. The outcome of the dispute was an agreement between the doctors and the government that resulted in major compromises on both sides and paved the way for the National Medical Care Insurance Act of 1966.

The development of the Canadian health care system can be viewed as a collaborative national endeavor based on values and expectations deeply rooted in the national character. These values and expectations were expressed initially by means of the Hospital Insurance Act (1957) and the National Medical Care Insurance Act (1966), and were reaffirmed in the Canada Health Act (1984). Essentially, these measures set up a framework for federal/provincial cost sharing of hospital and medical services, provided the provinces met specific conditions designed to establish and maintain certain national standards.

The standards on which the Canadian health care system is based are generally known as the five essential principles (Taylor, 1987, p. 441). The first principle is *universality*. This principle ensures that the same basic health care benefits are made available to all Canadians under the same terms and conditions.

The second principle, *accessibility*, provides for reasonable access to basic health services regardless of location. It is under this principle that user fees—in the belief that they impede access—are prohibited. Also, if basic health services cannot be accessed locally, this principle entitles Canadians to go elsewhere to receive them. Generally speaking, elsewhere has meant other Canadian locations, although in some instances—where a service, such as neonatal heart transplantation, was not available in the country—individuals have been allowed to go outside the country to obtain the service.

Third, all provincial medical insurance plans must provide coverage for a *comprehensive* range of health services, as specified in the Canada Health Act. These include, for example, care in complex academic medical centers, rural acute care hospitals, long-term, rehabilitation, and mental health facilities; community health services in urban, rural, and outpost settings; and air and ground ambulance transportation.

The fourth principle, *portability*, requires that coverage be provided to residents visiting other provinces as well as to those who have moved from one province to another and are awaiting coverage in their new home province.

Finally, the provincial health insurance plans must be *publicly administered on a nonprofit basis.* Many believe that it is this last principle that accounts for the significant cost differences between the health care systems in Canada and the United States. "If the universal coverage and single payer features of the Canadian system were applied to the United States, the savings in administrative costs alone would be more than enough to finance insurance coverage for the millions of Americans who are currently uninsured" (United States General Accounting Office, 1991, p. 3).

Benefits of Canada's health care system include medically necessary physicians' services, wherever rendered, and the services of other selected health professionals, such as physical therapists, chiropractors, and psychologists, generally under a physician's direction. Financing mechanisms vary from province to province, with the majority of provinces funding their programs from general revenues—British Columbia and Alberta excluded. In these two provinces, premiums are charged; however, in order to comply with the five principles of Medicare, exemptions are provided for those deemed unable to pay such premiums, either in whole or in part, on the basis of such factors as age and economic or medical status. In fact, the premiums provide only partial funding; the majority of financing comes through tax revenue.

Constraints and Challenges

Of the current issues capturing the attention of citizens in first world countries, health care is at the forefront. In the United States, President Clinton's task force on national health care reform has presented its health care reform plan to Congress. Great Britain has been in the throes of reformation of its health care system since its economic downturn in the 1980s. Among the western industrialized nations, the Canadian health care system is the only comprehensive system that has maintained a one-tiered structure providing services to all its citizens. The system is regarded as having much to offer those nations currently engaged in health care reform.

However, the maintenance of the Canadian health care system poses a significant challenge to individual Canadians and their governments in the increasingly turbulent and unpredictable economic climate of the 1990s. Because the universal health care system is highly valued by most Canadian citizens, any strategies undertaken to address the major issues must support the key principles of the system. Attention must be given to creating cost-effective, high-quality improvements that will allow the nation to sustain the comprehensive health care system to which it has become accustomed.

Public Sector Management. There are a number of constraints related to management in the public sector in general that must be addressed if the required changes in health care are to become a reality. Ring and Perry describe five such constraints: (1) policy ambiguity, (2) the relative openness of decision making, (3) a more direct and sustained influence from a greater number of interest groups, particularly the fund providers, (4) the need to cope with time constraints that are more artificial than those within the private sector, and (5) policy legitimation coalitions that are less stable and more prone to disintegration during policy implementation.

One of the two most distinguishing characteristics of the public sector, as described by Anthony and Herzlinger (1980), is the absence of a profit motive. However, while profit may not be a goal, cost containment and cost efficiency are of primary importance in the public sector. An organization's tendency to be labor intensive and to require relatively little capital per unit of output becomes an important consideration when cost and quality are at issue. Health care provides a vivid example of Anthony and Herzlinger's second distinguishing characteristic of the public sector—difficulty in measuring outputs. Although great improvements in output measurement are possible, considerable effort and funds must be expended to achieve them.

Finally, public organizations face difficulties in establishing goals and objectives since they must provide service as directed by an external body—namely, the fund providers. These constraints become magnified as new challenges are encountered and as costs increasingly must be contained.

Health Care Expenditures. Over the past several decades, Canada's health care expenditures have increased dramatically (Government of Canada, 1991). Initially, this growth was due to the introduction of universal Medicare. More recently, increases in health care spending can be attributed to (1) the expansion of the health care delivery system through the addition of new programs and services, (2) increased utilization of existing services, (3) increasingly sophisticated and expensive technologies, (4) a continual rise in consumer expectations, and (5) demographic changes.

The current and future outlook for the Canadian economy is not encouraging. For example, while the Canadian economy is expected to grow by 3 percent in 1994, unemployment is projected to remain relatively high, at slightly over 11 percent until 1995

(Conference Board of Canada, 1993). The level of national expenditure for health care is also cause for concern. In 1960, health care spending totaled about $2.1 billion ($120 per capita) and represented 5.5 percent of the gross national product (GNP) (Health and Welfare Canada, 1990). By 1987, total health care expenditure was $48 billion ($1,870 per capita) and 9 percent of the GNP (see Figure 1.1). In 1990, national health care expenditures had increased to 10.2 percent of the GNP (Health and Welfare Canada, 1993). Provincially, health care costs now account for approximately one-third of all government expenditures and a growing share of provincial GDP.

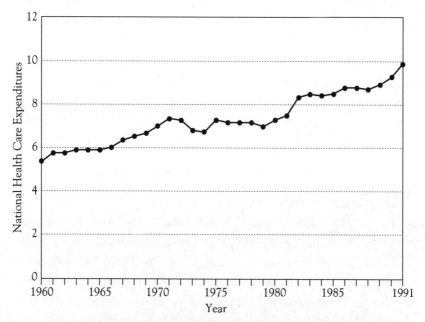

Figure 1.1. Total Health Expenditures as a Percentage of Gross Domestic Product, 1960 to 1991.

Source: Health and Welfare Canada, Health Information Division, Policy and Consultation Branch, May 1994.

Other Issues. Coupled with the slow economic growth and rising government deficits, there are other serious concerns within the health care arena. These include, for example, increasing tension between management and unions and competition rather than collaboration among various health care providers and health professional groups. There is also decreasing financial assistance by the federal government to the provinces (despite the fact that federal influence on the Canadian health care system was underscored in the Canada Health Act). The need for the provinces to manage their health care resources effectively and efficiently is growing increasingly urgent.

Over the past several years, both the federal and provincial governments have signaled a strong commitment to reinforcing accountability in all components and at all levels of the public sector, including the health care delivery system—to control costs, to ensure that the system remains viable and sustainable into the next millennium, and to set a vision that is understandable and that is shared by all stakeholders in the system. It is within this context that the University of Alberta Hospital exists and to these constraints that it must respond.

The University of Alberta Hospital

The University of Alberta Hospital is an 843-bed tertiary care academic medical center located in Edmonton. Situated on the campus of the University of Alberta, although autonomous from the university, it is the major specialty care and referral center for patients from northern Alberta, northeastern British Columbia, the Northwest Territories, and the Yukon Territory—a population base of about three million people in a referral area exceeding one million square miles. A full range of in- and outpatient services is provided in the newest of the hospital's facilities, the state-of-the-art Walter C. Mackenzie Health Sciences Centre. The Mackenzie Centre was constructed in the early 1980s, in the wake of several decades of prosperity in Alberta related to the oil industry. No expense was spared in offering to Albertans health care services as provided for in the Canada Health Act.

As Western Canada's major transplant center, the University of Alberta Hospital is involved in eye (cornea), kidney, heart, lung, bone marrow, and liver transplantation. Programs in trauma, cardiac sciences, neuro sciences, pulmonary medicine, and nephrology form the priorities for the organization. As well, the hospital is a partner with the Children's Health Center in the delivery of hospital care to children in Northern Alberta.

During the fiscal year ending March 31, 1993, the hospital admitted 30,313 patients, for a total of 319,806 inpatient days (University of Alberta Hospitals, 1993). At the same time, 388,524 outpatient visits (including emergency and day ward) were recorded and a total of 13,351 inpatient and 7,619 outpatient surgical procedures were conducted. The annual budget for the hospital is in excess of $290 million.

To carry out these activities, the University of Alberta Hospital employs a staff of approximately 6,000 people. About 350 academic specialist physicians are associated with the Faculty of Medicine at the University of Alberta. Complementing this large staff component is a major contribution from more than 650 volunteers. In addition, approximately 1,500 medical, nursing, and other students from a wide variety of health disciplines receive training at the hospital each year.

Not surprisingly, given their size and complexity, Canadian academic medical centers like the University of Alberta Hospital have been relatively resistant to change. Until quite recently, the changes that have been overtaking organizations in general, as well as those specific to the health care system, were far removed from the academic medical center environment. There was simply no imperative, funding or regulatory, for change.

Such is no longer the case. Academic medical centers are now finding themselves under increasing pressure to demonstrate clearly their unique value to the health care system as leaders in the provision of patient care, education, and research. Canadian academic medical centers now find themselves in the same position as other hospitals: change or be changed; proactively design and manage the future or have it imposed.

Addressing the Challenges

Increasingly, organizations are looking toward total quality management and innovation as the keys to meeting the rising demand for quality services with shrinking financial resources and for gaining some competitive advantage in an increasingly competitive marketplace. This is particularly evident in health care. As the hospital's chief executive, Donald P. Schurman, described during an interview for *Canadian Business Review* (MacBride-King, 1993, p. 6),

> In August 1992, the Conference of the Federal, Provincial and Territorial Deputy Ministers of Health brought together a group to articulate a new vision for the health care system. Out of that meeting came a statement setting out a vision of "a system which is consumer centered, providing the right service for the service receiver (the patient) by the right provider at the right time." . . . I would add another dimension, and that is "at the right cost," because I think the issue of cost is profoundly important for our health care system.

The hospital's executive group recognized that, while it could not control the environment, it was possible to manage it in such a way as to achieve a desired future for the organization. Perceiving that the health care system had evolved many systems, processes, and procedures that were of questionable efficiency and effectiveness, in relation to both waste and unnecessary cost, total quality management was viewed by the senior executives as an approach to deal proactively with these issues.

The implementation of total quality management began at the University of Alberta Hospital in 1990. At that time, the concept was diffusing slowly from American industry into the public sector. As more information about TQM and its potential benefits were acquired, it was recognized that the adoption of TQM as a fundamental management philosophy made a great deal of sense as a way to do business, including the business of delivering health care services.

It was also appreciated that the way care and services had been delivered in the past would result in expansion, increased utilization, and increased cost—a pattern that is no longer acceptable. For health care in Canada, this pattern would mean longer waiting lists, divisiveness and competition within and between organizations, rebellious taxpayers, challenging governments, disenchanted employees, skeptical unions, and harassed managers.

To create a different, more positive future at the University of Alberta Hospital, a new paradigm was needed. The years since 1990 have represented the implementation of that paradigm as the principles of total quality management have been introduced to the organization. Such a transformation is an evolutionary process with the potential to span almost a decade before complete and pervasive change can be acknowledged.

Over the past few years, however, many improvements have been realized, some of which will be addressed in subsequent chapters. Concurrently, from the broader system perspective, the economy has recessed and the funding of health care, as Albertans have come to appreciate it, is being compromised. In the early years of the 1990s, this funding, primarily from government grants, has not kept pace with inflation. Recently, actual cuts in the funding base have become a reality.

To address the financial challenge, much discussion has taken place regarding ways to restructure the health system in particular regions and throughout the province. At this point, it is unknown how restructuring will occur. It is expected, however, that these restructuring efforts may address some of the funding reductions as new systems of delivery are implemented throughout the province.

Total quality management has provided a concrete approach to the challenges associated with downsizing and elimination of waste and unnecessary care. Although there is much more to be accomplished, the commitment to total quality management has equipped the organization to proceed through difficult times. The capability of the organization to respond constructively to the changes required has been and continues to be markedly enhanced.

Through the experiences at the University of Alberta Hospital, other organizations may better understand the parameters, principles, and pitfalls associated with organizational transformation. They may be able to avoid the problems and benefit from the solutions and lessons learned as this one institution blazes the trail for other organizations to follow.

References

Anthony, R. N., and Herzlinger, R. E. *Management Control in Nonprofit Organizations*. Georgetown, Ontario: Irwin Dorsey, 1980.

Conference Board of Canada. *Provincial Outlook: Executive Summary—Autumn 1993*. Ottawa: Conference Board of Canada, 1993.

Government of Canada. *The Health Care System in Canada and its Funding: No Easy Solutions*. First report of the Standing Committee on Health and Welfare, Social Affairs, Seniors and the Status of Women. Ottawa: Government of Canada, 1991.

Health and Welfare Canada. *National Health Expenditures in Canada, 1975–1987*. Ottawa: Health and Welfare Canada, 1990.

Health and Welfare Canada. *National Health Expenditures in Canada: Summary Report, 1987–1991*. Ottawa: Health and Welfare Canada, 1993.

Health and Welfare Canada, Health Information Division, Policy and Consultation Branch, May 1994.

Hoffman, M. S. *The World Almanac and Book of Facts 1993*. New York: Pharos Books, 1993.

MacBride-King, J. "Prescription for Change." *Canadian Business Review*, Summer, 1993, pp. 6–14.

Porter, M. E. *Canada at the Crossroads: The Reality of a New Competitive Environment*. A report prepared for the Business Council on National Issues and the Government of Canada. Ottawa: Government of Canada, 1991.

Ring, P. S., and Perry, J. L. "Strategic Management in Public and Private Organizations: Implications of Distinctive Contexts and Constraints." *Academy of Management Review*, 1985, 10(2), 276–286.

Taylor, M. G. *Health Insurance and Canadian Public Policy*. Kingston, Ontario: Queen's University Press, 1987.

United States General Accounting Office. *Canadian Health Insurance: Lessons for the United States*. Report to the chairman, Committee on Government Operations, House of Representatives, Washington, D.C., 1991.

University of Alberta Hospitals. *1992/1993 University of Alberta Hospitals Annual Report*. Edmonton: University of Alberta Hospitals, 1993.

Chapter Two

Organizational Transformation: Positioning for the Future

Lynn M. Cook
Heather A. Andrews

The previous chapter provided an overview of the current health care system in Canada. As the evolution of the system continues, this current picture will become just a paragraph in history. There will be a new reality. What will it look like? That is not certain. However, there is no question that the challenges facing the system will be a strong force in shaping the future. For some organizations in the health care system, the lack of capability to harness the forces of change will result in a new reality that is unexpected and an organization that is ineffective.

It is the leaders in health care that will create powerful visions of a desired future and that will propel the system into that desired future. These leading organizations will have a framework for organization capability development that enables them to continuously reposition themselves, harnassing the power of change to make their vision a reality. Movement alone is not enough; winds of change blow in many directions. The movement must be coordinated and consistent.

Achieving the Vision

Imagine yourself as a member of a management team. Your team is on a plateau at the base of a tall, sheer cliff. Your mission is to stand on the upper plateau, high above your head.

To fulfill its mission of achieving the next plateau, the team has worked hard. You and your fellow team members have created a vision of standing there, observing the unprecedented view from the higher plateau. You have carefully developed a strategy for scaling the cliff. The team has purchased the best mountain climbing equipment money can buy. This new technology is touted to decrease by 30 percent the amount of time required to scale the rocky face. The team leader has hired a consultant who is an expert on cliff climbing. This consultant has created a new map of toeholds in the cliff face and has convinced the team that by using toeholds no one else has used before, the team will be successful in reaching the top, ahead of other climbing teams. And finally, the team members realize that they hold the key to success. They have undergone extensive physical training and mental preparation to develop into the most capable climbing team.

As you assemble your equipment at the bottom of the cliff, preparing for the climb, two people drive by in a pickup truck with a trailer. They stop, curious to find out what the team is doing at the bottom of the cliff. The team leader explains the mission to stand on the upper plateau. The two offer their encouragement and then hop out of their truck, unload their hot air balloon, and soon soar toward the mark. (The authors wish to acknowledge Jim Selman of ParaComm Partners International for the storyline.)

The people who manage the health care system are the climbing team. The cliff represents the challenges and forces of change facing the system. The upper plateau represents the health care needs of future generations. What is the shortest distance between the two points? Small incremental changes make the task extremely difficult and slow. As Albert Einstein said, "The world that we have made, as a result of the level of thinking we have done thus far, creates problems that we cannot solve at the same level at which we created them" (Bennis, 1989, p. 181). Rather, what is required is the ability to continuously reinvent organizations, making them capable of effectively using the forces of change to achieve desired results.

Organization Capability Development Framework

A strong, effective health care system is key to the health of citizens and thus to the strength of the society. As the needs and capabilities of societies change, so do the demands placed on the health care system. The leading organizations will be up to the challenge. The question is how to achieve the desired results.

History has shown time and again that people coming together in organizations can accomplish more than individuals working on their own. A health care organization is a collection of people. When one talks about transforming an organization, it must be recognized that corporations do not change—individuals do.

Organizational transformation is about each and every individual within an organization doing something differently, and it is about the collective change of individuals resulting in a difference for the organization. An organization able to continually change itself to achieve a vision unleashes within individuals the ability to truly do something that makes a difference. In addition, it coordinates that individual change. At the University of Alberta Hospital, the Organization Capability Development Framework has provided that coordination.

Organization capability is defined as the ability of an organization to continually reinvent itself in response to the challenges and forces of change facing it and to coordinate that action toward the attainment of its vision. It can be viewed as the composite of three domains: (1) the context, (2) the infrastructure, and (3) member capability (see Figure 2.1).

Context

The *context* is described as the components of the organization that create the environment within which activities take place. (It is important to recognize that the external environment exerts a significant influence on the organizational context. In this discussion of context, the description is confined to the environment within

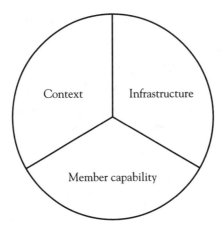

Figure 2.1. Organization Capability Development Framework.

the organization. This is an important delimitation of the term *context* as it is used here. The intent is not to diminish the importance of the external environment but rather to focus the discussion on the dynamics within the organization.) The objective of the leader is to create an empowering context—one within which people have the power to do the best they can in service to the customers of the organization. The components of the context include the mission, vision, values, principles, strategies, and objectives.

Mission. The corporate *mission* describes the reasons for which the organization exists. It typically outlines what value the organization provides to the people it serves. It also provides a frame of reference within which individuals within the organization can formulate their particular mission—that is, the specific value they provide within the organization in service to the corporate mission.

Vision. While the mission defines the purpose of the organization, a vision statement also forms a critical component of the context. Most effectively described in the present tense, the *vision* is an articulation of the preferred future of the organization as it fulfills the mission. Positioning oneself in the vision as if it were reality and comparing it to current reality enables the identification of the gaps that must be spanned for the organization to look the way it has been envisioned. As the desired future, the vision provides the focus to direct all present activity in a manner that moves the organization in a consistent direction.

Values. Corporate *values* create an understanding about the way in which people within the organization work together. Coordination of action is fundamental to organizational performance. That coordination is much more effective when people can anticipate the way colleagues come to the task.

Principles. A fourth important component within the context are *principles* to guide actions within the organization. The shortest distance between reality and the vision may be a straight line, a curved line, a zigzag line, or any number of other options. The best alternative may indeed be other than the straight line that represents the shortest distance.

Imagine the journey from today to tomorrow as going through a forest. There are many different strategies that could be applied, depending on the principles involved. If one principle were to minimize the destruction to the forest while moving through, a bulldozer likely would not be used. On the other hand, if one principle were to clear the way for others, a bulldozer might well be the ideal method to create the road.

Principles used as checks and balances for decision making bring consistency, which facilitates organizational change and increases the confidence level of organizational members. It is extremely useful for an organization to clearly articulate principles to guide activity and work within the organization. The principles become a reference point for all activity, work performance, and planning as the organization proceeds through the transformation process. As the principles become understood throughout the organization, they become important factors in enabling staff to measure their activities, actions, and proposals while moving toward the organizational vision.

Strategies and Objectives. The last components of the context are *strategies* and *objectives.* The former, with a longer-term viewpoint, signal a general manner in which the desired future will be created. Annual objectives with measurable results then drive the actions that cause the organization to move ahead.

The objective in articulating a powerful context for the organization is to create empowering mission, vision, values, and principles through which people have the power to be the best they can be in service to the customers of the organization. The context becomes personal to individuals as they create strategies and objectives to govern the work of their team and themselves.

Infrastructure

The next domain in the Organization Capability Development Framework is the *Infrastructure* (see Figure 2.1). The infrastructure is composed of the procedures and processes that exist in an organization and the systems within which work gets done. Procedures, processes, and systems are viewed in the framework as having three aspects: (1) technical, (2) relational, and (3) capability development (see Figure 2.2).

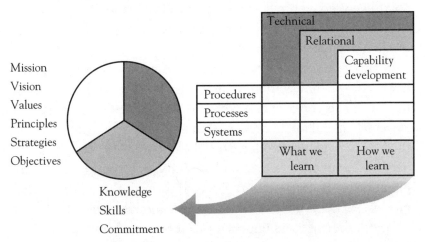

Figure 2.2. Organization Capability Development: An Integrated Framework.

Procedures, Processes, and Systems. *Procedures* link together to form *processes* and processes in turn link to form organizational *systems.* (For simplicity in the rest of the chapter, the word *process* will be used to refer to all three terms.) According to Juran (1974), current total quality wisdom suggests that 80 percent of quality problems that occur in organizations center around processes and 20 percent can be traced to people. Thus, fault finding and blaming when problems occur in the workplace may be misdirected and useless. The real problem may exist in the process itself.

Technical Processes. *Technical processes* pertain to the movement of materials, people, and information within the system. Many organizations have become very good at looking at their technical processes, applying quality improvement philosophy, tools, and techniques, and implementing changes that result in process improvement. But this focus on an organization's technical work is limiting. To truly transform an organization, there must be a recognition that the same discipline is required to improve the two other aspects of infrastructure: relationships and capability development.

Relational Processes. *Relational processes* are very different from those that focus on technical work. This component of the infrastructure is not about manufacturing or moving materials or information. It is not about delivering specific services. Rather, it is about the way in which people communicate and coordinate their actions in order to deliver products and services to the customers of the organization.

Too often, when interpersonal difficulties arise between people, common wisdom is forgotten. What are often referred to as "people problems"—communication difficulties, lack of commitment, errors or delays in accomplishing the work—are often evidence of relational process problems. The problems may stem from the lack of appropriate processes for coordinating action. This discipline surrounding the coordination of work with others transcends personal feelings and the "likability" of one's colleagues. Defining processes around how people relate channels energy toward achieving results.

A major system designed to support relationships is the organizational structure. It defines the primary reporting and communicating linkages. The intent to shift the focus of relationships can be actualized through a fundamentally different structure. For example, a functional structure promotes primary linkages to the department and secondary linkages to the customer. A change to a customer-centered design reinforces the importance of working closely with colleagues to deliver customer service, rather than to support a function.

Capability Development Processes. The third component of infrastructure focuses on *capability development processes.* Peter Senge (1990), in his book *The Fifth Discipline: The Art and Practice of the Learning Organization,* coined the concept of a "learning organization." How is it that organizations learn? It is not about a pile of bricks and mortar going down the street with a school lunch box. It is also not about "something in the air" in some organizations. Learning within organizations relates to the adoption of specific processes for capturing new learning and integrating it into the activities of the organization.

The objective in creating an enabling infrastructure for the organization pertains to the development of procedures, processes, and systems—technical, relational, and developmental—within which people can make their best contribution to the organization.

Member Capability

The third and final domain within the Organization Capability Development Framework is *member capability* (see Figure 2.1). Member capability pertains to the knowledge, skills, and commitment of the individuals in the organization (see Figure 2.2). The objective associated with member capability is the provision for people within the organization of opportunities to gain the capability needed to be the best they can in their work and in their service to customers.

Knowledge and Skills. Just as organizational change does not occur except as individual people change, improvements to corporate capability do not occur unless individual people become more capable. Within capability, people need *knowledge* and *skills*, not only about technical work, but also about developing and sustaining relationships and integrating new learning.

Formal processes to enable this capability development are needed. Effective performance management systems identify the capability needed for a position. Performance assessments reveal the gap between requirements and individual performance, enabling a focus on specific development needs. Capability development opportunities, such as orientation, in-service training, specialty training, conferences, and monitoring, are offered. Formal learning contracts with vigorous follow-up promote the integration of new learning into daily activities. This leads to improved individual, and therefore organizational, performance.

Commitment. Another important aspect of member capability is *commitment*. There are numerous examples of people who have knowledge and skills but are not committed to making the contribution they could make. Yet commitment cannot be taught. It is a personal decision made by each individual. This is where the power of the integrated Organization Capability Development Framework becomes apparent (see Figure 2.2).

Commitment is promoted in two respects. First, components within the context clearly describe what the organization is about and thus enable individuals to align themselves with the organization's purpose and vision and to understand how each person contributes to the future through day-to-day activities. Second, commitment is gained when people work within an organization in which the infrastructure is enabling rather than restrictive. Within the infrastructure domain, capability development processes enable each person to continually gain new knowledge and skills about technical work and the way in which people relate to each other.

It becomes clear that improvement in the capability of an organization depends on continuous improvement in context, infrastructure, and member capability domains. In addition, each of the domains must align with and reflect the principles and substance of the other. For example, one of the principles to guide decision making as set forth in the context may be empowerment and involvement. Unless the infrastructure specifically provides for such involvement and empowerment, the principle will not become a reality. And unless individuals are given the opportunity to become capable of taking charge of the work environment, "empowerment" remains just a word.

Organizational Capability Throughout the Organization

For the transformation of an organization to be successful, it must be led and strongly supported by the chief executive. However, if no one else in the organization changes his or her personal context, infrastructure, or capabilities, nothing will happen. Organizational improvement occurs through coordination of the activities of each and every member. Plans at the corporate level, no matter how well thought out, cannot drive change at every level. The Organization Capability Development Framework can be used to envision, plan, and implement this required coordination.

Consider the framework as a vertical cylinder with several levels (see Figure 2.3). Just as there is a corporate context, so the same elements exist at the departmental level. Each individual operating area requires its own mission and vision to describe how the area will serve its customers within the work of the organization. Although the area mission and vision must align with and complement the corporate context, they serve to reflect and amplify for individuals in the area their own reason for being.

The same analogy applies to the domains of infrastructure and member capability. From departmental mission and vision flow an area strategy and operating plan prescribing the specific activities that need to be undertaken. Departmental infrastructure and collective capabilities must reflect those described corporately.

Finally, the individuals within an area must have their own context, structures, and capability surrounding the specific work that is required. Even at an individual level, the framework can be used as a way of understanding, investing in, and designing the work that, cumulatively, moves the organization toward its desired future.

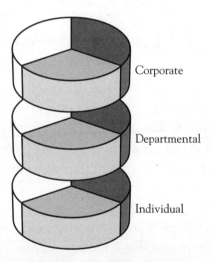

Corporate

Departmental

Individual

Figure 2.3. Organizational Capability Throughout the Organization.

Continuously Improving Organization Capabilities

One danger in describing an Organization Capability Development Framework for an organization is that it may be regarded as a static, one-dimensional structure frozen at a point in time. That perspective, of course, does not promote or support continuous improvement. The model comes alive when it is used to make deliberate changes in response to the desire to improve. This concept is illustrated in Figure 2.4.

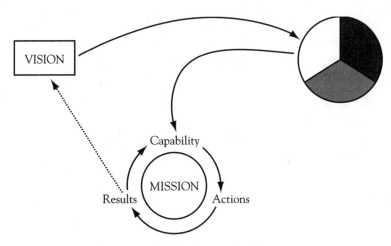

Figure 2.4. Creating the Future.

Applying the current level of capability, actions are taken and results achieved. The results are compared to the vision describing the desired future. For organizations that are committed to continuous improvement, the vision is always a step away. The gap that is created dictates the need to improve organizational capability and, in doing so, improve results.

The framework prompts review of the three components of organizational capability to ensure that the initiatives undertaken will result in breakthrough improvements. When results fall short of the vision, where are changes required? Perhaps, upon assessment, the procedures, processes, and systems of the infrastructure are judged effective and appropriate. The problem may be that people do not have the knowledge and skills to enable them to do their work effectively. That discovery would prompt a closer assessment of knowledge and skills. However, it may be that people do not understand or accept the vision. For organizational transformation to be effective, analysis of each domain and deliberate intervention where it is needed will lead to breakthrough results.

Change occurs when one person does something differently. Organizational transformation occurs with the coordination of the changes made by everyone within the organization. The Organization Capability Development Framework, used throughout the organization, focuses every action. It also prompts thorough review of each component for optimal intervention to achieve breakthrough results. This ability to focus and coordinate is what leads successful organizations to the achievement of a desired future.

References

Bennis, W. *On Becoming a Leader*. Reading, Mass.: Addison-Wesley, 1989.

Juran, J. M. *Quality Control Handbook*. Wilton, Conn.: Juran Institute, 1974.

Senge, P. M. *The Fifth Discipline: The Art and Practice of the Learning Organization*. New York: Doubleday, 1990.

Chapter Three

Organizational Alignment: The Framework in Reality

Heather A. Andrews
Donald P. Schurman

Throughout the organizational transformation associated with the commitment to and implementation of total quality management, the Organization Capability Development Framework (described in Chapter Two) has become increasingly valued at the University of Alberta Hospital for its clarity and its utility in focusing on and understanding particular components of the organization. As each of the domains was considered and developed, the framework assisted in assessing the alignment of the various components of each domain and of the organization as a whole. As each component was brought into alignment, a coherence was achieved as the organization moved into the new paradigm created within the vision.

It is beneficial to consider separately the domains and components within the organization in order to identify and address specific areas requiring improvement. At the same time it must be recognized that, in a complex system such as a hospital, such separation is artificial and can be misleading. In reality, each domain and component is interrelated and overlapping; changes in one must be reflected deliberately in the others. Otherwise, the organizational transformation will falter.

The Commitment to Total Quality

By 1989, the senior management team at the University of Alberta Hospital was well aware that a different approach to management of the health care system was necessary. The decision to commit to a total quality management philosophy, however, was not made lightly nor quickly. The issues that forced recognition of the need to change related to the constant demand for the provision of additional health care services with increasingly limited funds. The experience of total quality management in the private sector suggested that it was possible to increase the quality of the service or product offered while reducing costs and creating an empowering work environment. The philosophy appeared to be an ideal prescription for the ills that increasingly plagued the health care system.

The process of gaining commitment to this management approach started with the senior management team. Recognizing that such an initiative must be led from the top, a three-day retreat was held, which concluded with a strong commitment on the part of senior management to begin the change process. Soon after, the board and medical staff leaders were introduced to the concept; their response was generally supportive. The outcome of the process was a board policy statement setting forth the necessary support. While the board did not have a comprehensive understanding of the transformation that would be required in the organization and its culture, its policy statement was critically important.

The most challenging group to enroll—middle management— was the next point of dialogue. Through a couple of retreats, the general philosophy and implementation framework were reviewed. Although sufficient endorsement was received to begin implementation, a number of skeptics chose to "sit on the fence" to see how this change effort would unfold.

The middle management of any organization is a unique component in the process of organizational transformation: these managers are expected to facilitate change for the organization while at the same time undergoing major personal transformation. This was a significant request to make of middle management especially since it was indicated that the new philosophy would result in considerably fewer management jobs. Despite this, the degree of support from this group in many instances exceeded expectations.

As department-specific implementation plans were developed, they were guided by a corporate plan that delineated particular expectations and provided consistency in approach. Although this method was extremely useful in the early stages of transformation, it needed to be relaxed as staff became more expert in using the tools and techniques of total quality management. It was at this point that the utility of the Organization Capability Development Framework became apparent.

The Framework Applied

As was described in Chapter Two, the Organization Capability Development Framework is a valuable tool in developing and aligning the various domains and components of the organization during a transformation process. Described in the following section are specific initiatives that were taken at the University of Alberta Hospital to enable the organization to function on the basis of total quality management principles. Each domain with its relevant components is addressed.

Context

The *context* was described in Chapter Two as the cultural nucleus of the organization. Consisting of five major components—mission, vision, values, principles, strategies, and objectives—the context refers to the delineation for the organization of its reasons for existence, the direction it is headed, and how it is going to reach its destination.

Mission. An organization's *mission* is a description of its "reason for being"—that is, the value it provides to the people it serves. The mission of the University of Alberta Hospital (see Exhibit 3.1) is the result of extensive deliberation by the board, the senior administration, and the medical staff. It was developed as a reflection of the hospital's commitment to high-quality patient care and to the responsibilities for education and research associated with being an academic medical center.

Exhibit 3.1. Mission Statement of the University of Alberta Hospital.

Our Mission

The University of Alberta Hospital is committed to providing exemplary patient care and education in an atmosphere of compassion and scholarly inquiry while preserving the dignity and rights of patients and their families.

To meet the needs of those individuals entrusted to its care and to fulfill its obligations as an academic medical centre, the University of Alberta Hospital will:

- offer a wide range of patient care and health promotion services essential to the community and the region, including the development and delivery of highly specialized tertiary care programs;
- advance the health sciences by working in partnership with the University of Alberta and other institutions of learning to develop and carry out educational programs in a variety of health disciplines;
- promote, conduct, and apply research in association with the University of Alberta and other agencies for the advancement of patient care;
- pursue and manage its resources effectively and respond to opportunities and changes in the health care system with boldness and innovation;
- adopt a leadership and collaborative role with other health care providers in developing health care programs and assessing the health care delivery system; and
- generate a positive working environment that motivates staff and volunteers, fostering the productivity, pride, and well-being of both the individual and the organization.

The first portion of the mission statement embodies the essence of the organization. The balance defines the unique role of the hospital within the provincial health care system. An attempt is made to convey the ideal that the hospital's staff is the most important resource in meeting its mission. In addition, it is recognized that the organization has a responsibility to the public to obtain and manage shared resources responsibly.

Vision. In the process of organizational transformation, the *vision*, or the "preferred future," of the organization becomes a significant vehicle through which the commitment of members is created and sustained. Although the corporate vision is expressed by the senior team, there is recognition that the power in this description comes from its influence on the departments and individual shared visions throughout the organization.

Senge (1990, p. 13) uses the analogy of a hologram to enhance understanding of "shared vision":

How do individual visions come together to create shared visions? A useful metaphor is the hologram, the three-dimensional image created by interacting light sources.

If you cut a photograph in half, each half shows only part of the whole image. But if you divide a hologram, each part, no matter how small, shows the whole image intact. Likewise, when a group of people come to share a vision for an organization, each person sees an individual picture of the organization at its best. Each shares responsibility for the whole, not just for one piece. But the component pieces of the hologram are not identical. Each represents the whole image from a different point of view. It's something like poking holes in a window shade; each hole offers a unique angle for viewing the whole image. So, too, is each individual's vision unique.

When you add up the pieces of a hologram, something interesting happens. The image becomes more intense, more lifelike. When more people come to share a vision, the vision becomes more real in the sense of a mental reality that people can truly imagine achieving. They now have partners, co-creators; the vision no longer rests on their shoulders alone. Early on, when they are nurturing an individual vision, people may say it is "my vision." But, as the shared vision develops, it becomes both "my vision" and "our vision."

The vision statement presented in Exhibit 3.2 was developed by the executive team at the University of Alberta Hospital to communicate to staff the direction in which the efforts of the senior officials were committed. Departments, in turn, were asked to develop their own visions in alignment with and complementary to the corporate vision. As a description of the desired future, the vision statement provides direction to present activity such that the organization moves in a consistent direction. In addition, the importance of personal vision is recognized. Unless personal commitments and vision are compatible and aligned with departmental and institutional visions, a dissonance evolves that compromises the ability of the organization to make the transformation.

Exhibit 3.2. Management Vision Statement for the University of Alberta Hospital.

The University of Alberta Hospital:
A Leader in Creating the Future

The University of Alberta Hospital is a "value driven" organization where respect, partnership, and continuous improvement are demonstrated through our decisions and our behaviors. Staff, working in teams, and their unions are empowered and committed to constantly improving services to patients and their customers.

All staff display a deep sense of ownership and commitment to the issues and challenges faced by the Hospital. This results in a high sense of respect, excitement, and love of work as activities to celebrate the accomplishment of staff are seen constantly throughout the organization.

The dedicated knowledge, skills, and commitment of the most able hospital staff in Canada are manifest in delighted patients who display a deep sense of confidence and security as they entrust themselves to the care of the Hospital and the people who work here.

The exemplary performance of the hospital, as illustrated by breakthrough improvements, in key quality indicators and unheard of financial performance, is recognized throughout the world in research papers and numerous annual visits by world health care leaders who wish to directly experience the hospital learning organization. Performance data are continuously available to patients, the public, government, staff, researchers, and other health care providers.

The hospital is a highly sought after expert partner by governments, academics, unions, suppliers, and other providers as Canadians demand an improved, environmentally responsible and sustainable health care system. The findings generated by the Hospital serve as a map for the re-design of the health care system.

Values. Stated *values*, as a component of the domain of context, communicate to the organization members the desirability and importance of particular qualities and behaviors within the organization. By framing organizational activities in terms of these qualities and behaviors, expectations are created for the atmosphere in which work will be accomplished.

Early in the hospital's transformation to total quality management, the board and senior team ratified for the organization three values: respect, partnership, and continuous improvement. "Respect" was chosen to convey a valued attitude toward human and material resources. Staff, patients, and customers within and outside the organization as well as health care resources, would be treated with care, concern, and esteem. "Partnership" was intended to communicate the commitment to working effectively with staff, unions, physicians, faculties, government, and suppliers. The term chosen to convey the commitment of the hospital to management of quality within the organization was "continuous improvement."

Over the years that these values have been in place, they have been referred to frequently as an anchor and guide with respect to many aspects of hospital operation. They have been helpful in conveying organizational intent to patients. Most importantly, they enhance coordination of action by allowing people to anticipate the responses of their colleagues in the work situation on the basis of shared expectations.

Principles. As presented in Chapter Two, the *principles* delineated in an organization specify the concepts intended to guide action within that organization. They are used as checks and balances for decision making and thus bring consistency that facilitates organizational change and increases the confidence level of the organization.

At the University of Alberta Hospital, the commitment is "to deliver the best patient care available, to teach others to provide similar care, and to look for new ways to deliver care in the future" (University of Alberta Hospitals, 1993). To this end, seven principles of operation have been specified: (1) effective relationships, (2) empowerment and decentralization, (3) accountability and teamwork, (4) measurable, observable results, (5) process management, (6) customer satisfaction, and (7) collaboration.

Establishing and maintaining effective relationships is one of the key principles typically associated with total quality management. Effective relationships with partners, both within and outside the organization, are essential in accomplishing anything together and in achieving results in a manner that people experience as empowering. To this end, significant understanding has been achieved in relation to the processes surrounding effective relationships and, in turn, communication. Based extensively on the work of Business Design Associates (1991), principles fundamental to effective relationships and teams have been adopted. (See Chapter Four for discussion on rethinking the fundamental assumptions traditionally presumed to influence relationships.)

Empowerment is defined as having (or having access to) what is needed for fulfilling one's commitments within a defined role. *Decentralization* represents a commitment to promote decision making at the most appropriate point in the organization. Based on the belief that the organization's strength and potential rest with those who work in the organization, there is a recognition that the highest-quality decisions are made by the individuals most directly involved in the work. (Empowerment and decentralization as developed through a governance model in nursing and its subsequent evolution are addressed in Chapter Five.)

The principle of *accountability* suggests that no one individual is ever capable of knowing enough or of single-handedly controlling complex organizational processes. Recognizing that many different people in many different roles are necessary to accomplish the work of the organization, it is therefore crucial that members be able to count on one another. The notion of accountability is described as "count-on-ability"—that is, people must be held accountable for what we are counting on them to do.

With this notion of accountability, *teamwork* becomes vitally important for the success of the organization. Teams of people must be aligned in a manner that enables them to efficiently and effectively perform the work that the organization depends on them to do. (The principles of accountability and teamwork are addressed in Chapter Six in which organizational restructuring and resource allocation processes are explored.)

Management effectiveness is dependent on a disciplined focus on *measurable, observable results*. Evaluation of outcomes is essential if staff are to have the information they need to intervene skillfully in the design and management of effective processes.

As was mentioned in Chapter One, one of the distinguishing characteristics of public sector enterprise is difficulty in measuring outputs of the system. Considerable effort has been invested in creating systems to measure and respond to variability and outcomes of clinical care at the University of Alberta Hospital. (The processes associated with this endeavor are described in Chapter Seven.)

It is recognized that results are produced as a function of the processes existing in the workplace. The principle of *process management* is predicated upon the understanding that the creation of a different future or different results involves changing organizational processes and practices. Thus, two types of process change have been identified. First-order change seeks to stabilize and refine existing processes within a system. Fundamentally more important, second-order change seeks to break through historical levels of performance by making changes in the system.

Within the commitment to process management, there is a growing appreciation of the distinctions among the various types of processes and a recognition that all processes are not the same. Some processes facilitate coordination of action and satisfaction of customers. These are relational or "people" processes. Other processes (material or technical) pertain to the movement of materials, people, and information within the system and enable minimization of waste and maximization of efficiency. Capability development processes facilitate and promote the integration of new learning within the organization. (Process management is addressed in Chapter Eight, in which the alignment of processes associated with performance management is explored.)

Customer satisfaction is a principle that consistently appears in any discussion on quality management. The desires, needs, and opinions of the suppliers of a service or product are not satisfactory parameters for the well-informed, highly educated, and discriminating consumer of the 1990s. Organizations committed to quality management recognize and respond to this important understanding.

Customers, in the hospital's case, are not only patients, the ultimate consumers of the product or service, but also the staff and suppliers involved in complex interrelationships throughout the institutional operation. All those associated with the organization must be cognizant of the requirements and requests of the customers to whom they relate. Their ultimate goal must be customer satisfaction.

The principle of customer satisfaction is explored in Chapter Nine. The initiative addressed in that chapter is the redesign of the care delivery system within the hospital—an extensive project that is expected to encompass a review of all facets of the hospital's operation.

Coordination is an important aspect of people's relationships with one another. Work can only be truly effective through *collaboration* among those involved, whether on a project, on a team, or on an organization-wide basis.

Collaborating means listening to and, if appropriate, acting on the concerns and contributions of others in the course of accomplishing the work. It does not mean consensus or universal agreement. Rather, collaboration means involvement and inclusion of others in the design and coordination of work.

Within the hospital's complex environment, there are many stakeholders or partners in the process of providing health care to the patients who access the services of the organization. (Chapter Ten describes the importance of effective collaboration in these partnerships.)

Strategies. *Strategies* delineate direction for the organization during a certain period of time. The strategic plan articulates activities and sets priorities for action within the specified time frame. Within each department of the organization, strategies assist in aligning departmental action with the mission and the vision of the hospital and serve to delineate details of the organizational strategic plan. As with Senge's hologram analogy, the various strategies employed throughout the organization together create a complete picture of the organizational direction from a variety of points of view.

In 1991 a strategic plan was created for the hospital that set forth both clinical and operational priorities for a four-year period (University of Alberta Hospitals, 1991). Clinically, five program priorities were identified: cardiac sciences, trauma/emergency, nephrology, neurosciences, and pulmonary medicine. Operationally, the commitment to total quality management as a management philosophy was emphasized, as were a number of other related initiatives.

Each department—collaboratively and with multidisciplinary involvement—is expected to create its own strategic plan to demonstrate how it will align with the mission, vision, and strategies of the hospital. Although much is yet to be done, many departments have formulated their plans, and these have been reviewed by the hospital board.

Objectives. As staff members come to understand and appreciate the context being created, they develop personal periodic *objectives* with measurable results that enable them to align with the mission, vision, values, principles, and strategies of the institution in fulfilling their organizational roles. For example, all management personnel within the hospital participate in an annual process of setting goals with measurable results, each of which aligns with management competencies that have been delineated to reflect the context being created for the organization.

Infrastructure

The domain of *infrastructure* within the Organization Capability Development Framework was described in Chapter Two as the procedures, processes, and systems that exist within an organization and through which work is accomplished. A distinction was made among technical, relational, and capability development processes.

Technical Processes. As was noted in Chapter Two, through total quality management tools and techniques, many organizations have become effective in implementing change related to technical process improvement. *Technical processes* pertain to the movement of materials, people, and information within the system.

In the hospital, the preadmission process; the diagnostic process; and the processes surrounding delivery of supplies, medications, and meals to the patient are all considered technical processes. The time taken to document what has occurred to a patient while in hospital is also an illustration of a technical process related to information.

The complexity of an academic medical center is evident in the abundance and the complicated nature of the technical processes that are in place. Focusing on specified processes in an effort to eliminate waste and unnecessary activity often reveals that technical processes have burgeoned to contain many steps that add no value to the outcome. (Chapter Nine explores the redesign of care delivery and illustrates an approach to reengineering the technical infrastructure as it relates to delivery of care and services to patients.)

Relational Processes. *Relational processes* are associated with the ways in which people communicate and coordinate their actions in order to deliver products and services to customers. The work done by Business Design Associates (1991) has been increasingly appreciated within the hospital as a framework through which to assess the effectiveness of relational processes. (This fundamental understanding of relationships is explored further in Chapter Four.)

Another aspect of relational processes involves the formal structure of the organization. For hospitals, and perhaps for academic medical centers in particular, the traditional structure is an autocratic hierarchy formulated according to disciplinary functions and clinical services. With the commitment to working in teams and decentralizing decision making, it became apparent at the University of Alberta Hospital that the functional boundaries were inhibiting the ability of individuals to work collaboratively on process refinement. Budgetary allocation aligned with the structure, and so the responsibility and accountability for expenditures were not necessarily aligned with the source of a particular activity. For example, laboratory and radiology examinations were ordered by physicians in particular clinical departments, yet the budgetary accountability for this resource rested with the Laboratory and the Radiology Department.

To rectify the problem and bring the organization into alignment with the context that was being created, a change in the organizational structure was instituted. The focus of the change was to create relationships that were fundamentally different from those that had existed in the past and in so doing promote a more natural alliance among the staff who are accountable for particular groups of patients. The new structure was defined as a decentralized patient services structure. Three vice presidents were allocated to head up patient services teams. To the extent possible, all resources and staff directly associated with the relevant programs were assigned to these teams. Centralized services would be charged to the three areas on a negotiated price basis. Two other vice presidents assumed responsibility for corporate development and corporate support—services that would continue to remain centralized by virtue of their encompassing or uniquely specialized responsibilities. This formal organization structure is illustrated in Figure 3.1.

Figure 3.1. University of Alberta Hospital Organization Chart, June 1993.

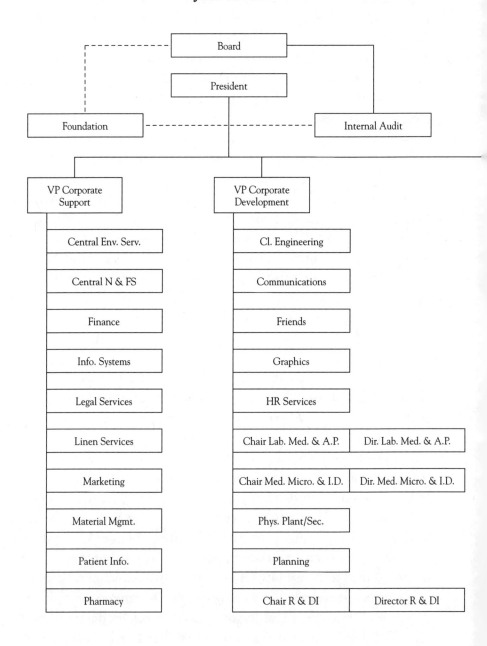

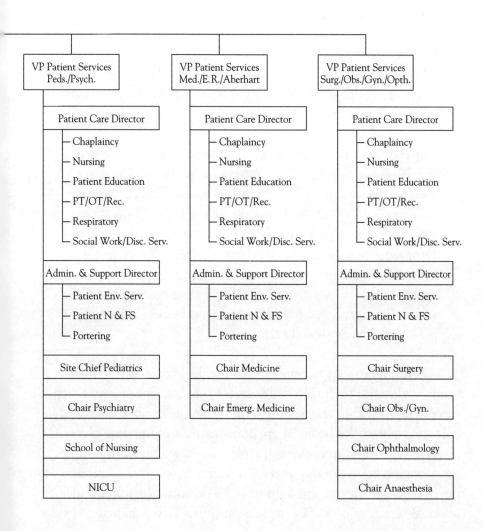

Capability Development Processes. *Capability development processes* were described in Chapter Two as the processes within the organization that relate to capturing new learning and integrating it into the activities of the organization. Based on Senge's (1990) concept of "the learning organization," there has been a commitment within the University of Alberta Hospital to continually assess the manner in which the organization is responding to change—that is, to continually improve the way in which improvements are made.

One event that illustrates this commitment was an invitation, subsequently accepted, to Dr. Don Berwick to visit the hospital. In addition to presenting a talk to the staff, Dr. Berwick was asked to assess the implementation of total quality management within the organization. Following his visit, Dr. Berwick wrote the chief executive of the hospital:

> I am extremely impressed, also, by the eclecticism of your learning style. You have spared no efforts, it seems, in locating resources and ideas for you to draw upon, and you have assembled these outside perspectives with flexibility, inventiveness, and independence. In so doing, you seem to have established a direction free from vows to a particular guru, using the talents of many helpers, and building an appropriately customized version of the changes you seek. Such search patterns and creativity, I think, have characterized the most effective journeys into improvement in other industries (D. Berwick, personal communication, 1992).

This commitment to using the best features of available theory, frameworks, and technology illustrates the concept of capability development within the infrastructure of an organization. Individuals throughout the hospital are continually seeking new ways of understanding and improving the manner in which work is done. As new paradigms are discovered, if they align with the organizational context, they are brought into the organization for consideration. When employees perceive the utility of such paradigms, they begin using them immediately. Thus the organization is continually learning and continually expanding its capacity to transform.

Member Capability

As was described in Chapter Two, *member capability* pertains to the knowledge, skills, and commitment of individuals within the organization. Employees and those associated with the organization must have the ability to do what they are being asked to do by the organization. At times of transformation, it is important to ensure that, if people do not possess the capabilities required, opportunities for appropriate development are provided.

Knowledge and Skills. *Knowledge* and *skills* are resources that individuals bring with them to their roles. In a hospital, there is a wide spectrum of expertise. The staff members of an academic medical center are among the most highly educated and most knowledgeable work forces of any organization. However, this knowledge typically is narrowly focused in a particular clinical or academic discipline and thus does not necessarily guarantee effective participation in an organization that is dependent on collaboration and teamwork for its success, both in the performance of specific job tasks and in process improvement.

In addition to the highly educated work force, many participants in a hospital setting have limited formal education and have been prepared "on the job" for the roles they fulfill. These people, too, require new knowledge and skills to enable them to work effectively with others to improve the way in which work is performed.

The University of Alberta Hospital is extensively committed to the capability development of its members. Programs to date have focused on the capabilities associated with the transformation to total quality management: working effectively with others; working in teams; employing the principles, tools, and techniques associated with quality management; and exhibiting quality performance in clinical utilization. Many staff members have availed themselves of the opportunities provided for skill development and have reportedly benefitted from the experience and knowledge they have gained. Of utmost concern within an environment committed to total quality management, however, is the notion of continual improvement of work processes. All members of the organization must be committed to and comfortable with consistently looking for ways to become more efficient and effective in their work while at the same time improving the quality of the service they deliver to their customers.

Commitment. *Commitment* of people within any organization also exists on a continuum. At the University of Alberta Hospital, the foundational beliefs about people form the basis for the emphasis on the development of member capability. The following quotation pertaining to beliefs about people is taken from the hospital's management statement (University of Alberta Hospitals, 1993):

- Diversity of our people is one of our greatest organizational strengths.
- Every individual cares about and is fundamentally committed to having our organization work for everyone—patients, staff, and other stakeholders.
- People are responsible; trustworthy; capable of choice, commitment, and mature/appropriate behavior. We all want to have our contribution(s) make a difference.
- Every individual has the capacity for continuous, lifelong learning and creativity in the face of today's rapidly changing reality.
- In order to get work done, we must coordinate our work with others. This coordination can only occur through the relationships we create and sustain with others. We can create the relationships necessary to carry out our work.

Recognizing that the decision to be committed is a personal choice, there are ways in which commitment can be promoted and encouraged within the organization—such as involving staff in the creation and description of a shared vision for the organization as was mentioned earlier. Total quality management encourages commitment through the implementation of such principles as empowerment and decentralization, collaboration, and partnership. In addition, an enabling infrastructure must be in place to promote effective and efficient linkages and teamwork. And, of course, people must be capable of doing what they are being asked to do.

Reflections on the Framework

Attention to the three domains of organization capability development can create a unified and aligned approach to organizational transformation. Recognizing that there is much to be accomplished and that progress occurs one step at a time, the framework as it is articulated for the organization provides direction for individuals, teams, and departments as they initiate change in their particular realms of responsibility.

It must be appreciated that, although the three domains of context, infrastructure, and member capability have been separated for purposes of consideration and description, such segregation is artificial. In reality, the domains and their components are interrelated and overlapping. Changes that are made in one domain must be reflected in the others. Where this is not accomplished, the dissonance will interfere with organizational transformation rather than promote it. Nevertheless, the Organization Capability Development Framework has been of great assistance in clarifying and distinguishing initiatives undertaken within the hospital and helping to ensure that the systems and processes within the organization are complementary and aligned.

References

Berwick, D. Personal correspondence. 16 October 1992.

Business Design Associates. *Offering New Principles for a Shifting Business World.* Emeryville, Calif.: Business Design Associates, 1991.

Senge, P. "The Leader's New Work: Building Learning Organizations." *Sloan Management Review,* Fall 1990, pp. 7–23.

University of Alberta Hospitals. *Strategic Plan—1991–1994.* Edmonton: University of Alberta Hospitals, 1991.

University of Alberta Hospitals. *Management Statement.* Edmonton: University of Alberta Hospitals, 1993.

Part Two

Principles of Total Quality Management

In the University of Alberta Hospital's implementation of total quality management, seven key principles were identified: (1) effective relationships; (2) empowerment and decentralization; (3) accountability and teamwork; (4) measurable, observable results; (5) process management; (6) customer satisfaction; and (7) collaboration. Part Two of this book is devoted to an exploration of the meaning of these principles in practice.

Each of the next seven chapters deals with an individual principle and describes its application within the organization. Although specific initiatives have been selected to provide illustration, it must be recognized that each of the principles has applicability in virtually all situations. Separation of the principles for discussion purposes is not intended to suggest that they function in isolation. Rather, they are viewed as complementary and significant in every interaction and initiative that occurs; indeed, they are regarded as the essence in practice of an organization committed to total quality management.

Chapter Four

Effective Relationships: Rethinking the Fundamentals

James C. Selman
Heather A. Andrews

The preceding chapters presented an overview of the thinking about and the approach to affecting transformation within the University of Alberta Hospital. As discussed briefly in the last chapter, it is axiomatic that nothing that has been or can be done is possible except within the context of authentic and effective human relationships. In any organization committed to total quality, relationships are necessary to get work done. Indeed, the ability to build and maintain congenial, warm relationships and to network effectively with people is one of the key competencies expected of personnel within the organization.

Nearly all of the early methodologies and models of change management assumed that the human dimensions of the organization were central, but they offered little if any guidance for focusing deliberate and rigorous attention on these dimensions. Various "people-sensitive processes" were tried, and some provided uplifting and positive team-building experiences. All, however, seemed to lack sufficient theoretical or intellectual rigor to be sustainable and applicable to large numbers of people over long periods.

It was recognized that, if the objective of organizational transformation were to be achieved, a method for distinguishing between generating principles and explanatory principles was required. For example, it was understood that "trust" was critical. What was needed was a way of *producing* trust, not simply a better under-standing of why it is absent or of how people justify not trusting management and one another.

By no means does this understanding alone result in a utopian state with respect to relationships. It is necessary to work daily on relationships within the institution. In fact, as the vision and com-mitments grow, so do the relationship breakdowns. This is both inevitable and healthy—an indication that the real underlying pat-terns and negative behavioral mechanisms are beginning to surface. These mechanisms normally are concealed, buried in bureaucratic resignation; they often thwart the best intentions to change. When they are uncovered, breakdowns in relationships are no longer taken for granted or covered over with platitudes. Rather, practices for getting to the bedrock question of what constitutes a "good rela-tionship" begin to develop—that is, what are an individual's com-mitments, and how can one learn to develop and continuously improve effective relationships?

Relationship issues in the hospital are inseparable from com-munication issues, and in most cases are the same thing—like heads and tails of the same coin. We are all familiar with the conventional wisdom, clichés, and folklore concerning these two crucial dimen-sions of organizations. However, practices for developing relation-ships and committed communication equal to the vision for the hospital of the future have not been evident. Until the total quality management journey commenced, individuals never had to con-front the deeper personal and philosophical questions that histori-cally had limited their capacity to think creatively and *design* relationships.

This chapter is based on the original, leading-edge work of Dr. Fernando Flores and his organization, Business Design Associates. The hospital was introduced to this philosophy and new practices by James Selman, a longtime associate of Flores and president of his own company, ParaComm Partners International.

What Is a Hospital?

In the context of this discussion, the first question might be "what is a hospital?" In posing this question, the ultimate definition or even the "right" answer is not sought. Rather, what is required is a response that can provide a way of observing the organization so that new possibilities for invention and design are created. For example, one can observe a hospital (like any enterprise) as being a group of human beings relating with each other and coordinating action together for the sake of producing a common future.

Modern Western hospitals are largely descended from the efforts of three individuals: Florence Nightingale, who organized nursing and made it a dignified profession with a high esprit de corps; Louis Pasteur, who developed the germ theory; and Joseph Lister, who applied Pasteur's germ theory. Without the contributions of these medical pioneers, plus some important nineteenth-century developments in anesthesia, surgery as it is now known would be virtually impossible.

The historical significance of these and other developments in medical technology is obvious. Less obvious is the fact that the models, structures, and practices for management of hospitals also grew out of the past—and many have not changed since the nineteenth century. Current management philosophy and associated practices have their origins in the military, where a command-and-control style makes sense. When change occurred very slowly (as it did prior to the middle of this century), people had few options; a control-and-procedure–based orientation to management worked reasonably well.

In the environment in which hospitals exist today, however, change is not constant, and it is accelerating in virtually every field. Complexity in organizations and systems is generally regarded as a primary source of anxiety and stress in the people responsible for their operation. In spite of management fads and twenty years of sophisticated information technology, our basic context for hospital management remains one of attempting to control human behavior in order to optimize the performance of tasks and procedures through the exercise of authority. Just as conventional surgery has changed with the advancement of medical and pharmacological technologies, so must traditional ways of viewing jobs and working together be examined in light of advances in the fields of human communication and management.

Relationships and Communication

Traditionally, hospital design emphasized the physical facility, the organizational structure delineating roles and authority, and finally, the information and materials processes that define the procedures and tasks to be performed. While they are all important, none of these aspects of design focuses on how people will communicate with and relate to one another, or provides a basis for integrating the hospital's design with its overall vision and commitment to patient satisfaction.

To address this concern, it is necessary to examine the fundamental interpretation of "who one is" as an individual and as a community. One must also inquire into the self- and culturally imposed limits on personal action and responsibility that in turn determine the boundaries for what is and is not possible in the future. Success in realizing intentions is accomplished through relationships with others. The future is continually being created through conversations with others—by asking for or making commitments, by making requests and promises. Any potential future exists only as a possibility unless and until it is realized through action. From this perspective, commitments are actions. Successful coordination in relationships is the coordination of commitments expressed in speech acts (Flores, 1982).

If one observes how people reach agreements about what is important, what is meaningful, and what does or does not work, it is evident that they do so by making assessments and assertions. Given our ordinary common sense, most people believe their assessments to be accurate descriptions of reality. All arguments and most right-wrong struggles are anchored in this view. While more difficult, it is more useful and empowering to consider assessments and assertions as speech acts, which can also be seen as commitments to an *interpretation* of "the way it is," not a matter of absolute fact.

All conversations occur against a background of commitments focused on either the past, the present, or the future. This view offers a new interpretation of interactions that occur within the organization and provides previously unseen possibilities for observing and coordinating human action in the institution.

The first challenge is to develop the basic competencies to observe, communicate with, and relate to others within a context of commitment. Then, the next challenge is to redesign the organization and work processes so as to enable people to navigate effectively in their network of relationships within the institution.

A New Discipline for Management and Design

Human beings coordinate action in the context of their relationships and through a process described as committed speaking and listening—conversation. For example, when a physician fills out a form to have a laboratory procedure performed, information is not merely being sent to another department. Rather, a request is being made of someone to satisfy some *condition of satisfaction* within some specified *time frame*. The physician will be satisfied if the accurate result is delivered within the required time frame. The technology and skill of a technician are strictly a means to this end. The physician is a customer asking for a service, and the technician is a performer promising to satisfy the conditions of satisfaction of the request.

Successful coordination requires that both parties understand and agree to this basic relationship. The job will not be complete until the physician/customer is satisfied. Failure to produce satisfaction results in resentment, resignation, and loss of trust, and it eventually reinforces a mechanistic, procedure-based, control-oriented organizational culture. Human beings cease being possibilities for one another and, more often than not, become "the problem."

Figure 4.1 depicts this basic structure, which is implicit in every situation or process in which coordination between two or more human beings is occurring. This is termed the *basic action workflow process*. These concepts and processes constitute the minimum and necessary distinctions for the design of any process or the development of new management practices for coordinating action within the enterprise.

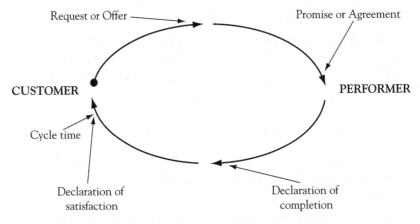

Figure 4.1. Basic Action Workflow Process.

The basic action workflow process diagram can be considered a map of the basic structure for observing the coordination of action among people. This representation, developed by Flores, is universally observable and is a constitutive aspect of all human enterprise. It proposes that nothing intentional occurs until someone initiates a request or an offer to have some condition of satisfaction fulfilled.

A condition of satisfaction is the criterion for satisfying a commitment of the person making the request or offer. It is important to note that a condition of satisfaction is always implicit in any request or offer and is usually interpreted in a context of shared traditions and practices. For example, if one requests a cup of coffee in North America, it goes without saying that the conditions of satisfaction include that it will be hot and black, unless milk or sugar is specified. In another culture, such as France, the implicit condition of satisfaction for the same request will include milk or cream.

In any workflow, there are always two roles. One is the customer whose conditions of satisfaction are to be met, and the other is a performer whose commitment is to satisfy the customer. After the customer makes a request or offer (which is an observable speech act), the customer and the performer negotiate until the performer makes a promise to satisfy the customer's conditions of satisfaction or agrees to the offer. Using this structure of interpretation it becomes evident, for example, how often people in the hospital make requests or offers assuming acceptance when in fact such agreement has not been reached. By focusing on explicit speech acts or commitments in each phase of the basic action workflow process, ambiguity, misunderstanding, and subsequent breakdowns are significantly reduced or avoided altogether. Further, when miscoordination occurs, it is a relatively straightforward matter to analyze its cause and make a correction.

Upon reaching agreement, the conditions of satisfaction are produced by the performer. This phase is completed by a declaration—another speech act—in effect saying, "The job is done." The coordination, however, is not complete until the customer also declares, "Yes, you met my conditions of satisfaction. Thank you." Unless or until all of these core speech acts are accomplished, there will be uncertainty, potential dissatisfaction, and waste accompanied by the sorts of interpersonal tension, upset, and moodiness that are all too commonplace in organizational relationships.

The basic action workflow process represents a simple act of coordination. In actuality, all of the institution's processes are made up of many workflows having many customers and performers. What has proven invaluable is having a common language and the same structure of coordination at many levels—from the institution's overall relationship with its patients, to the intermediate processes by which a patient is satisfied, to effective individual coordination within a unit.

Observing work in this way is very different from simply viewing work as a series of procedures or activities for controlling the movement of material or information. Not only does this structure allow organizational members to understand the conceptual framework of human coordination, it also allows them to observe waste from a new perspective.

Waste occurs for a variety of reasons and takes many forms. In contemporary society, waste is viewed mostly in physical and material terms. Organizations generally attempt to reduce it with technology and increasing levels of organizational complexity. This often leads to even greater levels of wasted effort and creates a kind of "downward spiral" in which the more improvement is attempted, the less it is actually realized. More importantly, in enterprises such as hospitals, in which most of the work is service oriented, this approach to the elimination of waste fosters bureaucracy and self-justifying practices.

For example, it is frequently alleged that physicians drive up the cost of health care by requesting many tests and procedures that are not clinically necessary. Attempts to deal with this belief administratively have included adopting new policies, control systems, committee review processes, training, and sometimes outright pleading. Yet most professionals agree that this remains a source of significant waste and expense in many institutions.

Why do attempts to effect this kind of change fail in spite of general agreement that it is a problem and that change is needed and beneficial? One suggestion is that people have misinterpreted the problem and are therefore attempting to effect solutions that not only do not make a difference, but often produce more problems and negative morale.

Rather than viewing the problem as "unnecessary procedures," consider the possibility that the problem is a lack of coordination and trust among the various participants in the institution, combined with insufficient commitment to clarifying and fulfilling the conditions of satisfaction for a particular request. From this perspective, one can begin to see waste as an opportunity to build relationships and to bring forth innovation, commitment, and clear communication.

Waste occurs whenever people are unclear about conditions of satisfaction or about their commitments in the relationship, when a basic action workflow process is incomplete, or when roles become confused. This waste takes the form of delays, confusion, dissatisfaction, breakdowns in relationships, and unnecessary or redundant actions.

Committed Communication

All communication involves speaking—whether orally, in writing, or through some electronic medium. It also involves listening. Listening is not the passive "hearing" of information. Rather, it is active and interpretive, based on the competencies, historical background, culture, and commitments of the people involved in the conversation.

In the human networks that comprise organizations, it is obviously crucial for people to speak and understand the same language. Just as people in a hospital need to share linguistic distinctions relating to health care technology, it is equally important that they share basic distinctions for the effective coordination of action in day-to-day conversations. Five basic linguistic distinctions through which all human coordination takes place are highlighted in Flores's work (1982): assertions, assessments, requests, promises, and declarations.

Assertions

Assertions are defined as statements made by a speaker as fact that can be witnessed or verified by a third party. The commitment of the speaker is to provide evidence if asked. An assertion can be true or false but can always be verified through independent observation if challenged (example: "We are $X below budget.").

Assessments

Statements made by someone that are an interpretation for the sake of furthering action or opening new possibilities are termed *assessments*. When made responsibly, assessments are always specific to some domain of action, relative to some standard, and may or may not be supported by assertions or facts. Assessments can be agreed to by others but ultimately are neither true nor false. The commitment of the speaker is to offer grounding for the assessment if asked (example: "We can improve the quality of our services.").

Requests

Requests are commitments that require that some action be performed within a particular time frame; they are always associated with some condition of satisfaction. A request is not a want or a desire. It demands some response in the form of acceptance (a promise), a decline, or a counteroffer (example: "I request that you do this job in less time with the same resources starting next week.").

Promises

Promises are commitments to perform some action that has been requested. An unsolicited promise is an *offer* that is conditional on being accepted by someone else. Promises may be revoked, in which case the person revoking the promise must be responsible for the consequences of this action and its effect on his or her relationship with others or, in some cases, by paying compensation (example: "I promise to implement the change by next Saturday and will advise you when it is complete.").

Declarations

Declarations are speech acts made by those who have been granted authority to speak on behalf of some community of people. Declarations are commitments that become possibilities and/or facts in the moment of speaking (example: "I pronounce you man and wife.").

With these basic distinctions, people learn to proactively listen for opportunities to coordinate more effectively, and they are also able to observe instances in which coordination is breaking down. Moreover, new questions such as "why are we having this conversation?" begin to displace older habitual responses, such as having to justify and defend a point of view.

Committed speaking and listening is not a panacea, nor is it necessarily comfortable. It does, however, provide a basis for surfacing and resolving breakdowns quickly, for building relationships and trust, and for observing how human beings coordinate commitments. This interpretation does not replace the need for effective management of materials and information systems, but it can greatly simplify their design and implementation.

Lessons Learned

As the concepts and processes of committed speaking and listening became increasingly understood by individuals within the University of Alberta Hospital, the power of the new conceptualization surrounding effective relationships was apparent and valued. Of particular benefit were the concepts associated with (1) the basic action workflow process, (2) the importance of conditions of satisfaction, (3) the value of negative assessments, and (4) the principles of effective relationships.

Basic Action Workflow Process

The *basic action workflow process*, as a framework for understanding human interaction and relationships, made an important contribution to the understanding of how work is accomplished and what elements are required to further action associated with the work. By appreciating that every interaction oriented toward the accomplishment of work is initiated by requests or offers, conversations between individuals became very focused. People began to ensure that each of the elements was addressed and clear and that discussion was purposeful and centered on the request or offer. Once this aspect of the interaction was clearly understood by both parties, subsequent action to accomplish the task became much more fruitful and productive.

For example, the basic action workflow process became an important consideration in discussions surrounding labor and management relationships. In situations involving a union grievance against the actions of the employer, once the circumstances surrounding the incident had been described, it became very productive to clearly understand the request that the union was making. In the past, meetings had often concluded without a specific understanding of the actions that could be taken to resolve the issue. By focusing on the request from the union's point of view or the offer from management's point of view, it was possible to effectively negotiate a solution that would address the alleged problem. From there the solution would be implemented, a declaration of completion would be made, and a response from the union would be anticipated.

Through attention to the basic action workflow process, relationships surrounding the accomplishment of work have become more productive and effective. Individuals have become conscientious about understanding requests and ensuring that specific commitments requiring attention are assumed by specific individuals and that each person agrees to fulfill the particular action.

The Importance of Conditions of Satisfaction

A second concept that has demonstrated significant utility in ensuring effective relationships has been described as *conditions of satisfaction*. As defined earlier, conditions of satisfaction arise in the continuous conversations between customers and performers as they coordinate action. They serve to clarify the outcome(s) to be produced when the action has been completed. In mutually developing an understanding, both customer and performer can be responsible for ensuring that there is satisfaction and alignment throughout the process.

In an organization responsible for delivering health care to patients, it is very important that caregiver and patient *mutually* determine the conditions of satisfaction associated with the patient's experience with the organization. In discussing the care available to the patient, caregivers should understand as clearly as possible what the patient's expectations are, recognizing that the objective is patient satisfaction whether the expectations can be made explicit or not or whether they change through time. For example, the patient may expect to have the linen on the bed changed every day. However, that may not be possible in an organization that is attempting to be effective and efficient in its use of supplies. It may be possible, however, to negotiate with the patient that the sheets will be replaced when they are soiled but otherwise they will be straightened and reused. Such an understanding at the outset of an encounter may avoid disappointment and dissatisfaction later on in the hospitalization.

Conditions of satisfaction, when articulated as part of *any* request for or offer of action, enhance clarity and mutual understanding in the relationship between the customer and the provider.

Mutual understanding and a commitment to continuous co-invention of the conditions of satisfaction assists in the elimination of delays, confusion, dissatisfaction, breakdown in relationships, and unnecessary or redundant actions.

The Value of Negative Assessments

In a culture practiced in indirect, tentative, defensive, and adversarial communication, *negative assessments* are frequently viewed as uncomfortable, impolite, harsh, and unproductive. In light of the previous description of assessments, the understanding that negative assessments represent an interpretation for the purpose of furthering action or opening new possibilities is very productive. Assessments, whether negative or positive, are neither true nor false—they are simply one's interpretation of a situation. They may be grounded in or supported by assertions, or they may not. The power associated with the concept of assertions, however, comes with an understanding of the value of negative assessments.

Typically, the response to positive assertions is inertia; it is good to know that perceptions of situations are complimentary, but the outcome is usually "more of the same." It is when people seek to understand and respond to negative assessments that there is a potential for change. Negative assessments open the door for further exploration of situations and creativity surrounding ways to address matters from new perspectives. When team members feel they have permission to make negative assessments, the potential for advancement and creative change is markedly enhanced.

Consider a situation in which a supervisor is conducting a performance interview with a subordinate. During the discussion, the supervisor observes, "It is my assessment that you are having difficulty setting priorities and keeping your calendar commitments under control." This negative assessment could provide an opportunity to explore observations that ground the assessment: "You are frequently late for meetings or miss meetings that you are scheduled to attend." "You appear to be out of control and continually in a panic." "I have received complaints that you are not empowering the people you work with and insist on being involved in every detail." These observations could then lead to a discussion of ways in which the problem could be addressed.

By requesting honest assessments from colleagues, individuals can progress significantly on an ongoing basis. The realization that negative assessments provide valuable feedback assists the organization as a whole in progressing effectively toward the required transformation.

Principles of Effective Relationships

Closely associated with the processes of committed speaking and listening are *principles of effective relationships*. These have proven exceedingly valuable, both in informal conversations in the workplace and in the more formalized settings associated with meetings and small group interaction. As these principles are continually reinforced as ground rules for conversation and interaction, the effectiveness of relationships is markedly enhanced.

The principles of effective relationships (Selman, 1991) are as follows:

- *Listen Generously*
  This means learning to listen for the contribution and commitment of the other person and suspending assessments, judgments and opinions about what they are saying. This does not mean that we agree or disagree with what is being said, but that we are committed to the legitimacy and value of their view.

- *Talk Straight*
  This means speaking honestly in a way which forwards the action as opposed to reacting to or attacking what is being said. This includes learning to make clear and direct requests.

- *Be For Each Other*
  This means believing in and committing ourselves to the premise that we are all in this together and that no one individual can win at the expense of another. This is the basis for trust and for making it safe for each other to take risks without fear of censure or being undermined by one's colleagues.

- *Honor Each Other's Commitments*
  This means respecting each other's commitments, including one's own.

- *Appreciate and Acknowledge Each Other*
  This means that each member of the team commits to continuously acknowledge and appreciate the contributions of others and the team itself, even when things do not work out. It also means requesting and receiving acknowledgment from others if it is missing.

- *Be Concerned for Inclusion*
  This means asking the question, "Who else should be included or has a stake in what we are talking about?"

- *Be Concerned for Alignment*
  This means participating in every conversation with a commitment to build alignment. Alignment does not mean consensus or universal agreement. It means that everyone is either "committed to" or "able to support" the commitments of others. No one is committed against the direction we are moving.

These principles have been posted in all the meeting rooms within the hospital and have become part of every meeting agenda that is prepared. By continually referring to them as conversations are carried out, the efficiency and effectiveness of communication and relationship processes are maintained at a highly productive level. It has also served to facilitate the constructive discussion of difficult and potentially explosive issues.

As the organizational transformation has matured and evolved within the hospital, the importance of committed speaking and listening in every facet of the operation has been emphasized. The readiness with which individuals have incorporated the concepts into their daily activities attests to the relevance and utility of the framework.

It has become glaringly apparent that the principles of effective relationships have applicability in every facet of the organization's operation and are relevant to each of the other principles addressed and illustrated in subsequent chapters. The notion of committed speaking and listening is viewed as a previously missing ingredient in organizational change initiatives. Within the hospital, it is viewed as the primary catalyst that will enable the transformation to succeed.

References

Business Design Associates. *Offering New Principles for a Shifting Business World.* Emeryville, Calif.: Business Design Associates, 1991.

Flores, F. "Management and Communication in the Office of the Future." Unpublished doctoral dissertation, Department of Philosophy, University of California, Berkeley, 1982.

Selman, J. "Ground Rules for Effective Teams and an Empowering Organizational Culture." Unpublished paper presented at Banff Management Conference, Banff, Alberta, September 1991.

Chapter Five

Empowerment and Decentralization: A Model for Staff Involvement

Heather A. Andrews
Donald P. Schurman

Involvement of individuals in decision making is closely tied to the concept of democracy as it is valued in the industrialized world. Although many in the Western industrialized nations would claim to exist in a democratic environment, the extent of empowerment and decentralized decision making in the workplace typically does not reflect this value. As Ackoff (1989, p. 11) describes,

> Although most industrially advanced countries are committed to democracy in the public sector, most of their organizations—corporations in particular, but even organizations within government—are organized autocratically. The power to reject any decision made by individuals below the top level of most organizations is concentrated in the hands of senior managers. The explanation for this system is usually that hierarchy is required in organizations that must manage divided labour efficiently, and that hierarchy entails centralized control—autocracy—no matter how decentralized the organization.

This stance is increasingly being questioned as the power of total quality management in organizations is recognized and experienced.

The initiative described in this chapter was funded in part by a grant from the Alberta Health Job Enhancement Fund. Appreciation and acknowledgment are expressed—the involvement of staff in this process would have been difficult without this support.

The reshaping of our concept of democracy is firstly global in nature. The institutional impact can be viewed as a local manifestation of a much more pervasive phenomenon. It is suggested that the forces that are reshaping the economic and political maps of the world are also at play in redefining and restructuring Western hierarchical organizations and individual participation.

On the individual level, there is increasing recognition of the personal needs associated with feeling useful to others, being involved in solving problems, and being recognized and respected. DuBois and Lappe (1992) argue that democracy must be redefined in a way that allows citizens the opportunity to be involved in solving society's problems on an ongoing basis.

At the organizational level, the leadership of the University of Alberta Hospital is committed to involving members in defining and solving organizational problems. The beliefs about people as forwarded in Chapter Three call for empowered staff coordinating their actions to meet customer requirements.

Having made the commitment to the empowerment of staff and to provide for their involvement in decision making, it was recognized that a specific organizational structure was required to make this contextual commitment a reality in practice. The experience of the nursing organization in the hospital serves as an example of the development, implementation, and revision of a concrete mechanism to enable this to happen.

Shared Governance

Members of the nursing profession have been advocating the concept of "shared governance" for over a decade. Although a precise definition is elusive, those who address the concept refer to ideas such as shared decision making; collaborative governance; governing councils; participative professional practice; and professional accountability in regard to control, authority, and accountability. One of the primary proponents of the idea, Tim Porter-O'Grady (1987, p. 283), describes his view of the concept: "The goal in a shared or professional governance model is to determine the base of accountability for each functional service component and build appropriate structures" based on (1) assigned authority; (2) a managerial role to facilitate, integrate, and coordinate; (3) professional obligation for care and ongoing operation of nursing service; (4) self-supported and self-directed nursing care systems integrated with other patient services; and (5) assurance of standards of clinical practice. As Merker and Burkhart (1991, p. 2) describe, "In shared governance, decisions are collectively made at the unit level and are integrated at higher levels. Decision-making responsibility and accountability are distributed throughout the organization, and managers move from a leadership role to a facilitator role."

The major premises of the shared governance model hold that (1) the quality of decisions is much better when those who are involved in the front line operation, and thus are responsible for carrying out the decision, are involved in making it, and (2) commitment to implementation is greater when one has been involved in the choice of direction. The capability—knowledge, skills, and commitment—of all members is acknowledged to be one of the organization's prime resources. This chapter highlights the development, implementation, and revision of a shared governance structure in the Nursing Division of the University of Alberta Hospital.

Background

The Nursing Division of the University of Alberta Hospital had long been viewed as a traditional organization with the typical bureaucratic hierarchy associated with a large academic institution. With the imminent commitment to total quality management, steps had been taken to flatten the organization in an attempt to empower staff and decentralize decision making, but it was recognized that much more could be accomplished.

In 1988, the decision was made to recruit a new vice president responsible for nursing services. This person was charged with introducing changes over a two-year period to revitalize and renew the nursing organization. This period of change was viewed within the hospital as an opportunity to enhance the perspective and professional profile of nursing; full support was vested in the new vice president and in the initiatives proposed.

Among the many initiatives introduced by this change agent was a structure of shared governance. Based primarily on the framework proposed by Porter-O'Grady and Finnegan (1984), this organizational shift was among the first of about a dozen significant divisional changes instituted by the new vice president.

Early discussions with union officials brought that group to the table in support of the project. A Nursing Council was created that included both staff nurse participants selected by administrative personnel and union representatives. The shared governance structure was under way within a couple of months.

The initial governance structure consisted of the Nursing Council plus six committees that reported to the council. Each committee was composed of staff nurses representing the seven departments in the nursing structure plus selected resource personnel. In the early days of the functioning of the structure, much of the business was orchestrated by the vice president and brought to the Nursing Council members for ratification. Nevertheless, the staff felt as though they had significant decision-making capability since early successes generated changes in dress code for nurses and name tag designations—visible evidence of council activity in areas of concern for nurses.

The test of the model came in the summer of 1990 when a major financial cutback was called for in the Nursing Division. In the spirit of shared governance, the challenge was taken to the Nursing Council by the Vice President (Nursing)—now a different individual from the aforementioned vice president. The response of the council members to the request to eliminate a major portion of operating dollars was a refusal to participate. Stating that they could not be involved in decisions that might eliminate the positions of some of their colleagues, they directed the responsibility for decision making to the administration.

This challenge proved to be a crisis that had not been contemplated when the original governance model was developed. Ensuing months were fraught with problems, including (1) the union representatives and some staff nurses withdrawing from the council table, (2) great unhappiness about decisions relating to major cuts in operating funding, (3) a breakdown of communications between the union and the nursing administration, and (4) a general threat to the viability of the model.

It became evident that the shared governance model could not stand the test of a serious issue. There were, however, two major understandings that surfaced as a result of the crisis: (1) Because the implementation of shared governance had been rushed, insufficient process and planning had been involved in the adoption, development, and implementation of the change. (2) Nurses and management throughout the hospital rallied to support the concept of shared governance and were not willing to abandon it. Although there had been major problems with the initial implementation, all were willing to try again and address the shortcomings of the first endeavor.

Designing a Model of Governance

Once the commitment to redesign the governance structure was secured, the task of selecting members to participate in the process was undertaken. It was determined that membership for the developmental task group would be sought from throughout the nursing organization. Staff members were asked to indicate their interest in participating; as it happened, it was possible to involve all of those who offered. Participation was also sought from the two relevant unions (nursing professionals and paraprofessionals) and the various categories of the administrative structure in nursing.

The Nursing Governance Task Force began its work in the spring of 1991 by reviewing literature on shared governance and exploring models implemented within other institutions. Once the various designs were understood, the group concluded that it would be difficult to proceed with the task without revisiting the philoso-phy of nursing within the hospital. The philosophy was subse-quently revised with the involvement of and feedback from participants throughout the Nursing Division. The task force then undertook the task of articulating a mission and vision of nursing. These three contextual documents—the philosophy, mission, and vision statements—ultimately became a coherent foundation upon which to base decisions related to an appropriate governance struc-ture to promote individual empowerment and involvement in deci-sion making.

As the group members gained an understanding of the shared governance models described in the literature and "tried them on for size" in the context of the hospital, it was determined that the best route would be to custom design a model for the organization rather than to select one developed for another institution. As with the development of the nursing philosophy, mission, and vision, the creation of the governance model was accomplished through the use of tools and techniques associated with quality improvement. Initially, brainstorming was used to identify matters that require decision making in nursing. The individual decision tasks were clus-tered into relevant categories, and an encompassing description that captured the essence of all the items in each respective category was created. Through a process of discussion and refinement, these groupings eventually became the subjects of four divisional coun-cils: the Professional Council, the Practice Council, the Commu-nication and Informatics Council, and the Resource Management Council.

The model as it was developed is illustrated in Figure 5.1. The building blocks of the model were decentralized councils (center circle) with the patient/client as the focus. This was intended to convey the commitment to the care of the patient and the focus of nursing activity on the consumer of the care. The decentralized councils functioned as the local decision-making bodies, attending to matters arising within specific clinical practice areas.

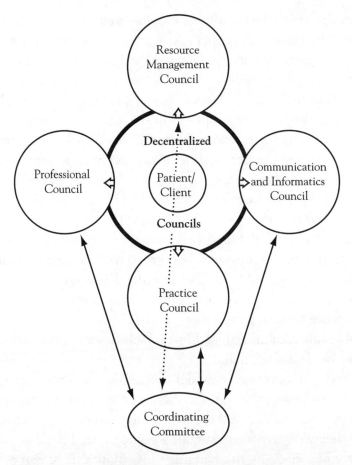

Figure 5.1. C.A.R.E. Model of Nursing Governance.

Each of the four divisional councils was assigned areas of responsibility. The Professional Council dealt with issues related to the
profession of nursing, work life matters, research and scholarly activities, and advanced practice roles, and was the resource group in
matters relating to the implementation and refinement of the governance model itself. The Practice Council dealt with matters relating to nursing practice and operations, including nursing protocols
and procedures, expanded nursing functions, and the assessment
of the quality of practice. The Communication and Informatics

Council assumed the coordination of liaison activities among nursing and the related disciplines and departments as well as information management matters as they related to nursing and clinical practice. This group also attended to communication of information within the Nursing Division. Resource matters, both fiscal and human, as they pertained to the delivery of nursing care were dealt with by the Resource Management Council. This group came to have a beginning understanding of funding systems, factors influencing the use of resources, budgeting, accounting, and other matters related to the effective allocation and use of resources.

Matters that did not clearly align with one of the divisional councils or that related to more than one council were discussed by the coordinating committee. This group had no decision-making role but was responsible for coordinating the activities of the four divisional councils and channelling information and issues in an appropriate fashion. Information among councils was shared at the coordinating committee meetings and subsequently communicated among divisional councils.

Once the governance model was developed for implementation throughout the Nursing Division, a contest to name the model was held. As staff received their orientation to the proposed structure, they were invited to submit a name for it. The final choice of title was made by the Nursing Governance Task Force. The name that was chosen was the C.A.R.E. Governance Model, an acrostic representing the first letters of the main principles underlying the model: Cooperation, Accountability, Responsibility, and Empowerment.

Implementing the Model

Implementation of the newly developed governance model began in the summer of 1992 and spanned a period of about six months. Initially, decentralized councils were formed primarily of units with similar patient populations and working with one nurse manager. As implementation of the model proceeded, decisions were made to combine decentralized councils to accommodate groups with similar issues and to provide for efficient use of resources. Each decentralized council provided one member to participate in each of the four divisional councils. In this way, communication with each area in the nursing division was direct and effective.

The divisional councils were activated in sequence with the Professional Council, the first to be functional. To help smooth the transition, several members of the Nursing Governance Task Force continued as members of the Professional Council to oversee implementation of the model as it was designed. The remaining divisional councils were activated at a rate of approximately one every two months. Where the nurse managers functioned as facilitators for the decentralized councils, the directors of nursing facilitated the divisional councils. The coordinating committee, consisting of the Vice President (Nursing) and the chairs of each of the divisional councils, served to channel information and issues but was not involved in decision making.

As the model was being implemented, much effort was invested in clearly describing the responsibility, authority, and accountability for decision making associated with the various groups. The implementation of the governance model in nursing did not mean that all staff were involved in every decision. An attempt was made to delineate what decisions were to be made by whom within the organization. One useful guideline stipulated that if the decision had impact on only one particular area, then the decision could be made at the local level. If another group was also affected, then representatives from that group were to be involved in the decision making as well. If the issue affected the Nursing Division as a whole, the matter would be dealt with by one of the divisional councils.

A number of decisions continued to rest with the management structure. In particular, those related to the hiring, firing, and disciplining of staff were viewed as inappropriate for delegation. The articles of the collective agreement also influenced the direction decisions could take and emphasized the importance of consultation with appropriate union and human resources personnel.

Much energy was invested during the implementation phase in acquainting council members with the issues and factors affecting particular matters. For example, the Resource Management Council devoted many initial meetings to educational sessions pertaining to budgetary process; achieving understanding about operating, capital, and special purpose accounts; and factors affecting funding allocations. In addition, it was necessary to provide members with the requisite capabilities for being involved in group decision making. Competencies for participating in groups, forwarding ideas, handling debate, resolving conflict, and effectively participating in meetings were included in the preparation of members for meaningful and empowered participation in the model.

After the model was fully implemented, the majority of the business of nursing was carried on through the council structure. As issues arose, there was commitment to collaboratively arrive at solutions. For example, in many areas staff were becoming involved in the recruitment and selection of new staff members. It soon became apparent that the process varied throughout the institution and that the collective agreement was not being applied consistently. A group of representatives from management, the union, human resources, and staff agreed to work on the problem. The outcome was a set of guidelines to direct staff in the process that pointed out the aspects that required careful attention and consistent application.

There were many instances of exciting and creative approaches to problem solving with respect to the model. The next section addresses process and outcome challenges associated with the initiative.

Outcomes of the Initiative

The implementation of the governance structure was not without its complications and concerns. The detailing of the outcomes is divided into two segments: challenges during implementation and status after a major organizational change.

During the Implementation Process

Several challenges became apparent as the implementation of the governance structure proceeded. One issue related to the role of the union as it pertained to the structure.

The Nursing Governance Task Force took the position that the decentralized and divisional councils would identify the resource personnel who could assist members in addressing the matters arising on their agendas. Some union representatives had a different understanding—that they would be guaranteed a seat on each of the councils. Although ultimately each divisional council chose to have as a member a representative from the union, there was distrust, discontent, and unhappiness while the decision process ran its course.

In the midst of the implementation of the divisional councils, a meeting was held with members of the decentralized and divisional councils in existence at the time. This meeting provided an opportunity to create an inventory of "What's working?" with the structure and "What's missing?" Recognizing that the various groups were in different stages of implementation, the following itemizes the successes and challenges at that point as identified by the participants.

What's Working? When nurses, both staff and management, were asked to identify the features of the governance model that were working well for them, they named as a major area of satisfaction the involvement of all in decision making. This was viewed as positive in that there was shared ownership of problems and solutions, issues were being taken seriously, and there was increased interaction among staff at varying levels of experience. In addition, increased commitment to the final decision was noted.

Commenting on the impact of the model within the practice unit, some staff identified increased collegiality among members and a "different" atmosphere as features that were working well.

Communication was clear, the global perspective was understood, and creative methods were being used to ensure that all received the information.

In terms of morale, staff members used terms such as excitement, increased involvement, input to change, increased control, and increased understanding to describe the positive impact participation in the governance structure was creating. Several voiced an increased appreciation of the importance of data in decision making and told of increased involvement in data collection in their areas of practice. One person stated that increased understanding of the content and significance of the collective agreement as a factor in decision making was a positive outcome. Many agreed that collaborative decision making and being part of the solution worked well in their areas.

What's Missing? In some cases, factors that represented positive features of the implementation in certain areas were posing problems in others. For example, where one group expressed appreciation for information encompassing the global perspective of hospital activity, another group felt that the global perspective was missing and thus detracting from its ability to be effective. The mechanics of the implementation presented a problem for a number of staff. In particular, the time commitment, the difficulty inherent in getting people together, problems of staffing in the absence of some caregivers, and the financial support required to permit participation posed extensive challenges for some.

Communication represented an issue in some areas in that staff identified problems in getting information to and receiving it from various segments of the organization. Others commented on "too much paper." There were concerns about the clarity of communication and the proliferation of the use of "jargon" throughout the hospital. Concern was also expressed regarding an understanding by front-line staff of the corporate direction of the hospital.

Another major issue related to education. There were concerns about overwhelming amounts of information, uncertain knowledge of the collective agreement, and the need for training in effective teamwork and meeting skills. Several members commented on the resentment of staff that were left to "do the work" when other staff members were off the unit participating in the governance structure: "We need to understand and appreciate that working on work is work."

Descriptors relating to the "mood" of the workplace were in evidence when talking about "what's missing." In addition to resentment of other staff and problems with the collective agreement, trust was identified as an issue, although the specific problems associated with this were not identified. A lack of enthusiasm surrounding the model was a concern for some, while others cautioned that they needed to have realistic expectations—that is, they needed to understand that a pervasive organizational change such as this takes years to become fully operational and effective and does not produce immediate results.

The need for further clarification of decision-making processes became apparent as the "missings" were discussed. Flexibility was advocated around the need to change decisions if indicated. Clear specification of the authority associated with the decision making was also stipulated. Finally, the need to evaluate the results of decision making was emphasized.

Evaluation of the outcomes of the model was initiated. The topic had become a major research initiative on the part of the Nursing Division, and a number of people became involved in the process on either a short- or a long-term basis. Not only was the model's effectiveness in assessing achievement of the goals of empowerment of staff and involvement in decision making being addressed, there also was an attempt to assess the cost-effectiveness of the structure. In fact, it was determined by Montgomerie (1993, p. 7) that for the implementation period (July 1992 to May 1993) the actual cost of operation (including education) of the governance structure was $284,857—approximately .1 percent of the hospital budget. The challenge associated with this assessment was to apply a price tag to the nebulous features of empowerment and quality of decisions.

Impact of Organizational Change

The C.A.R.E. Governance Model, having been fully implemented since January 1993, ceased functioning in August 1993. In June 1993, a significant organizational restructuring was instituted at the University of Alberta Hospital (this initiative is described more fully in Chapter Six). The typical disciplinary divisions of the hospital were eliminated, and interdisciplinary teams focusing on care for particular groups of patients were created. This meant that there was no longer a Division of Nursing.

Prior to that, concern about the cost of the model in terms of the release of staff to attend meetings of the four divisional councils had been becoming an increasing concern of both staff and management. (The survey to assess the actual cost of the model was mentioned earlier.) The Vice President (Nursing) made a request to the Professional Council, which was, in turn, relayed to the other three divisional councils, to plan for a 50 percent reduction in the cost of supporting the model.

Subsequent to the organizational change, another request was made that the Professional Council consider ways to make the structure interdisciplinary, particularly at the decentralized level, to ensure that it aligned with the new structure and that all disciplines and workers had an opportunity to be involved in relevant decision making. At the same time, the hospital was attending to a significant budget reduction that eventually led to the layoff of about 270 employees. Prior to that, about forty management positions had been deleted.

In the midst of this tumult, at a general meeting of the nurses' union, those in attendance expressed concern that the model was not being implemented as it had been designed. Some nurse managers were not perceived as effectively involving their staff in decision making. In addition, the requests being made by the Vice President (Nursing) were viewed as compromising the model as it initially had been developed—for nurses only. The union took the position that it would not support the model and advised nursing staff in writing not to participate.

In response to that advice, the chairs of the four divisional councils (at that time, staff nurses) met to determine how to respond. It was their decision to cancel all meetings until the issues could be resolved.

Subsequent discussions with the union resulted in an impasse: The union would not support the model unless it continued as it was originally designed—that is, for nurses only. The hospital could not support the structure if it remained applicable exclusively to nursing. There was a recognized need for a nursing advisory committee, and the organization continued to support and encourage that type of structure exclusively for the profession.

The Next Generation

Within the new organizational structure, the hospital remained committed to the empowerment of staff and the decentralization of decision making. However, interdisciplinary collaboration in decision making was also required.

The next-generation structure consisted of interdisciplinary participation on the patient care units. A specific structure was not stipulated; however, managers were expected to involve appropriate people in decision making related to the issues at hand. Each of the disciplines was encouraged and supported in the development of a discipline-specific professional council. As part of the process, multiple professional councils worked together to align terms of reference and determine how they, as professional bodies, fit into the structure of the organization.

Lessons Learned

Although the full implementation of the C.A.R.E. Governance Model spanned only about five months, there were a number of issues and problems that became lessons in the longer term. The following comments are based on a survey of costs of the model (Montgomerie, 1993), a December 1992 meeting of staff involved in the model, and feedback received by the Vice President (Nursing) during the development and implementation periods.

Parameters of Decision Making

A major challenge associated with implementing the model was defining the appropriate decision processes—that is, what decisions could be addressed by decentralized/divisional councils, what decisions were administrative, and what decisions had implications for the collective agreement and were thus, according to the union, "out of bounds." Some good work was done on this issue involving both union members and management, but there were still instances in which some staff felt that they should have input to and influence on every decision while others believed that parameters were required.

At the outset of an initiative such as the one described in this chapter, it is important to develop a clear understanding of decision-making parameters. Are *all* decisions open to input from staff throughout the organization? Do particular groups (unions, management, the board) have a designated responsibility for certain decisions? When input is sought, what will be the decision-making process? In answering these questions, the concept of levels of authority as described by Creative Nursing Management (1992,

p. 19) was particularly helpful. By designating levels of authority associated with each decision initiative, the ground rules were established from the outset. Staff were involved in the decision as to whether they would have full authority for the determination and implementation of a decision or whether their input and advice were being sought but the decision would be made by another group. By establishing such parameters ahead of time, it was possible to avoid disillusionment and disappointment when the process was different from that initially presumed.

Costs of the Model

The cost of supporting people in their attendance at divisional council and decentralized council meetings became an issue. In an era of fiscal restraint, many staff expressed concern about spending money on nonessentials (in their minds) when staff were being laid off. (As was reported earlier, Montgomerie [1993] determined that the amount required to support the C.A.R.E. Governance Model was about .1 percent of the operating budget of the hospital.) Staff also expressed concern about the number of people involved and the fact that these people required relief to attend the meetings of the councils. The following comments from the Montgomerie (1993, pp. 11–12) survey illustrate some of these concerns:

1. The concept of divisional councils in the C.A.R.E. Model is excellent. However, in these times of cutbacks and budget restraints, I find it difficult to understand how the hospital can justify paying 3 to 35 people per council for 8 hours once a month on 4 councils.

2. Although a progressive idea, the fiscal environment at present does not warrant the funding of such programs. I would prefer to see my colleagues and myself gainfully employed. What good is autonomy if few of us are employed?

3. I feel councils unnecessary at this particular time—decisions are made at the board level. Waste of time and money.

4. I feel that divisional councils are expensive, as are decentralized councils. However, I believe a good investment is being made.

In retrospect, the four-divisional council structure was expensive and cumbersome. In a time of fiscal constraint, it is particularly important to ensure that the organizational structures are streamlined and efficient. The cost of the C.A.R.E. council structure became prohibitive.

At the point at which the union took the position of non-support of the model, the Professional Council was considering ways to make the structure more cost-effective. With the new organizational structure, fewer decentralized councils would exist. This would diminish the number of representatives involved and thus cut costs. As well, there was a recommendation being formulated that the Professional and Practice Councils be combined. The shortening of meeting time was being considered, too.

Effectiveness of Councils

In the opinion of some staff members, no meaningful decisions were made during the functioning of the councils. Although this perception was not shared by all, it was of great concern that this was the assessment of any. The following comments (Montgomerie, 1993, pp. 13–17) provide a spectrum of observations about the effectiveness of the councils.

1. Are the councils, subcommittees, task forces making that much of an impact on the overall running of the hospital? Are the councils working on projects that Administration has already okayed and/or rejected, thus making councils' work redundant?

2. I am having trouble determining outputs of those large councils and am concerned about lost communication between councils, decentralized councils, and staff members not on councils.

3. Our hospital is supposed to be patient focused—the patient comes first? In general councils are okay, but in many ways a waste of time.

4. There is a concern that councils really have no decision-making powers. The majority of items coming to council are level I [data collection] or level II [formulating recommendations] authority. If this remains the case, cheaper methods of data collection and communication can be found.

Input relating to questionable effectiveness, particularly of the divisional councils, was proliferating. It was necessary to critically evaluate the "value added" by the divisional councils; formal evaluation of this aspect had not occurred because the life of the four-division council structure was relatively short. The new-generation structure was developed to ensure that the professional councils used efficient processes and formats to address the matters of concern to them.

Role of Union Representatives

The role of the union became an issue in the two implementations of a nursing shared governance structure. As the second implementation proceeded, it became evident that there were discrepancies in the understanding of where the union fit into the picture. Some members of the task force that developed the model believed that each decentralized and division council should determine its own requirements in terms of resource personnel. The union representatives believed that they had been promised involvement in every council. This discrepancy caused conflict throughout the implementation.

Involvement and support of the union is important to the success of a project such as this. However, it is imperative that all parties understand at the outset their involvement in the development and implementation of the model. It was the position within this organization that the participants in the model were the staff of the institution, with the union as an important stakeholder. The specific role of the union in the model was not adequately understood or discussed, nor did the union understand how its role in the organization needed to change in response to a philosophy of total quality management. (Partnership with unions is explored briefly in Chapter Nine.)

Role of Managers/Administration

As the model was created, the role of management personnel in the C.A.R.E. Governance Model was to facilitate the various councils throughout the organization. No provision was made for specific representation of management on the divisional councils, which resulted in that group feeling disenfranchised and alienated from the activities of the councils. Some of the comments from Montgomerie's (1993, p. 12) survey supported this observation:

1. Nurse managers' valuable input has to be obtained by going to their meetings since they are not members of councils.

2. Many of the institution's most expert people [nurse managers] have no avenue to participate in councils, and this concerns me.

3. Need all levels of nursing represented for differences in knowledge.

As the commitment of the University of Alberta Hospital is to provide an avenue for participation of all relevant individuals in decision making, the role that was created for administrative staff was untenable. Although in some circumstances the structure and process functioned well, in other areas the rigidity and legalism of staff with respect to the involvement or noninvolvement of their nurse manager interfered with the basic provisions of the new philosophy associated with total quality management.

When the councils ceased functioning, a process was under way to respond to a request from the managers for representation on each of the divisional councils. The lessons learned from dealing with this issue reinforced the need for a recognized and legitimate role for managers in the coordination and facilitation of action. The revised structure ensured that the administrative personnel within the organization performed appropriate roles within the framework while at the same time involving staff in decision making. (Chapter Eight describes a system to ensure that this is accomplished.)

Overlap of Council Activities

As business within the divisional councils proceeded, it became evident that there was overlap in the matters being attended to, particularly by the Professional Council and the Practice Council. As members commented (Montgomerie, 1993, p. 13):

1. There is repetition of information discussed at the different council meetings. This happens frequently, and I find that when I finally can bring "home" some concrete information to staff, it has already been discussed, which makes me feel that my role is useless.

2. Councils repeat efforts. Could be combined.

Recommendations to combine councils, particularly the Professional and Practice Councils, emerged. This was accomplished through the formation of a nursing advisory committee and other professional advisory committees. Concerns about overlap and duplication have since been alleviated.

Relevance of the Resource Management Council

With the organizational restructuring, the Resource Management Council became irrelevant since there was no longer a Division of

Nursing or a nursing-specific budget. Following the structural change, resource issues were dealt with by an interdisciplinary team at the program and patient care levels.

The Resource Management Council was an invaluable tool for acquainting staff with the processes associated with budgeting and operation within the hospital. However, with the new organizational structure, a nursing-specific forum to attend to budgetary matters was no longer relevant. In its short period of operation, it was not possible to assess the benefit or lack thereof of this particular council.

The hospital is committed to the empowerment of staff, decentralization of decision making, and interdisciplinary forums at the local level. The next-generation structure provided for this. As well, the development of an advisory committee for nursing supported and encouraged the involvement of nursing staff in decisions about professional matters.

The Issue of Trust

It was reported earlier that "trust" was identified as an issue in the assessment of "what was not working" with the governance structure. The specifics of the "trust issue" were never detailed, however. In trying to understand this problem, it became apparent that "trust" (or lack thereof) was a concept used throughout the organization in a careless and irresponsible manner; there was no obligation to specify the facts (assertions) contributing to this assessment.

In further exploration of the problem, the clarification provided by Business Design Associates (BDA) (1992, p. 11) became increasingly valued. BDA contended that the generalization of the term *trust* is not sufficient to assist with the forwarding of action or the resolution of problems. Rather, consideration must be given to three fundamentals of trust: competence, sincerity, and involvement.

Competence refers to reliable and competent performance. Did staff not trust that the structure and/or individuals were able (competent) to carry out the designated decisions or to involve them appropriately in decision making? *Sincerity* pertains to the intent or desire to honor or fulfill one's commitments or obligations. Perhaps the staff did not trust that management really was committed to involving them in decisions related to their work. *Involvement* relates to the commitment to include and consider the advice and opinions of stakeholders and customers in decision making. Involvement rests on a sufficient relationship based on mutually agreed upon and respected commitments. As described in Chapter Four, the relationship must demonstrate the fundamentals of effectiveness if interactions are to produce the desired results and be mutually satisfying.

As hospital members have continued to work on the disciplined understanding of "the trust issue," success in resolving specific matters has been enhanced. An increased understanding regarding the concept itself has assisted in this problem resolution.

The Hospital's Experience

The process of developing and implementing a governance structure within the hospital was a profitable and educational experience. It was helpful to understand and grapple with the issues that have emerged. This process is being regarded by the executive group of the hospital as an important step in the evolution of an institutional context that promotes a decentralized and patient-focused structure.

It is evident that changes within the health care system are ongoing, inevitable, and pervasive. The more extensively individuals within the organization are involved in decision making regarding their practice, the more effective will be the care offered to the patients. Through the commitment to true democratization of the workplace, the quality of care will be markedly enhanced.

References

Ackoff, R. L. "The Circular Organization: An Update." *Executive*, 1989, 3(1), 11–16.

Business Design Associates. *Morale, Trust and Partnership*. Emeryville, Calif.: Business Design Associates, 1992.

Creative Nursing Management. *Leaders Empower Staff* (course workbook). Minneapolis, Minn.: Creative Nursing Management, 1992.

DuBois, P. M., and Lappe, F. M. *Living Democracy: Overcoming the Myths That Control Us*. San Rafael, Calif.: Institute for the Arts of Democracy, 1992.

Merker, L., and Burkhart, E. E. *Shared Governance Models*. Chicago: American Hospital Association, 1991.

Montgomerie, H. *Report of the Cost Survey—C.A.R.E. Model*. Edmonton: University of Alberta Hospitals, 1993.

Porter-O'Grady, T. "Shared Governance and New Organizational Models." *Nursing Economic$*, 1987, 5(6), 281–286.

Porter-O'Grady, T., and Finnegan, S. (eds.). *Shared Governance for Nursing: A Creative Approach to Professional Autonomy*. Gaithersburg, Md.: Aspen, 1984.

Chapter Six

Accountability and Teamwork: Restructuring and Resource Allocation

Eric W. Taylor

Accountability and teamwork were identified in Chapter Three as key principles in the University of Alberta Hospital's implementation of total quality management. In that discussion, the complexity of organizational processes was pointed out, as was the inability of any one person to totally comprehend all factors within the organization that must be considered when a decision is made. The quality of any decision is enhanced when those involved in the activity or process under consideration are involved in its determination, be it related to patient care or to the allocation of scarce resources.

In this respect, there must be structures and processes in place such that people are held accountable for what they are "counted on" to do. As the University of Alberta Hospital executive group became more aware of the significance of this notion, it became apparent that neither the organizational structure nor the budgeting process promoted this principle.

Background

One of the major measurement systems employed in organizations revolves around the comparison of actual operating results to operating plans. Deviations from anticipated performance results often give rise to what is termed *variance analysis* and should lead to some sort of management action either to change the operating plan or to redirect action to get the organization back on track. Since this variance analysis assumes that the budget is an appropriate plan, the budget process is clearly an important facet in every organization.

The budget represents a formalized allocation of organizational resources to achieve defined goals. It is the operating plan translated into financial language. The budget communicates to the members of the organization the relative importance of the various components and activities. Through the delegation of budget responsibility to individuals, some control by individuals over organizational resources is indicated—a reflection of the responsibility structure. Once that structure is set, budget allocations make clear the amount of control individuals have over the resources they need to achieve their performance goals.

With this in mind, the organizational structure becomes an important aspect of the infrastructure in regard to the budget since it is the alignment and relationships provided in the organizational chart that tend to signal the need for accountability and teamwork surrounding the resource allocation decisions made within the operational areas. The organizational structure also indicates the amount of participation and coordination that will be required in other areas in which staff do not have complete control over resources needed.

In government circles, the process of budget allocation is the essence of the political discussion. Wildavski (1975, p. xii) makes this point in discussing the political power created in budgeting: "Budgeting is so basic it must reveal the norms by which [people] live in a particular political culture—for it is through the choices inherent in [allocating] limited resources that consensus is established and conflict is generated." Budgets become signals: They become a process through which organizations and their members attempt to direct the activities of others.

The Budget Game

Consider the following images, which were created by organizational members trying to describe the old budget process: (1) driving a car by looking in a cracked rearview mirror, (2) a poker table with "Donny the Dealer" (Donny being the chief executive) making deals under the table, (3) a dinner table where some have more than enough and others do not have enough to sustain themselves, (4) periodic airlifts dropping extra resources into the operation in a period of crisis.

These were the perceptions of members of hospital management in 1991 when discussions of changes in budgetary process first began. At that time, a large number of people were led through a process of envisioning images to describe the current budget system and the budget system they were looking for. The then-current budgeting process was viewed as unfair; it was seen as not rewarding the appropriate individuals and did not support the strategic needs and goals of the organization, and it focused little if any attention on long-term strategic needs. And since it had grown up in the context of government funding, it was built around the concept of "incrementalism." That is, budgets in the new year were based on the previous year's experience plus or minus some small adjustment factor but without serious or extensive review of past operational activities. At one point, in a time of plentiful provincial resources, it had even gone so far as to rely on "last-dollar financing," which allowed an organization to overspend its resources in any particular year and be bailed out at the end of that year by the government.

Now, contrast those images with the following: (1) an organization that is driven by looking to the future rather than to the past, (2) an organization where all come to the dining table and leave with enough to sustain themselves, (3) an organization that demonstrates fairness and proactiveness in responding to community needs. These were the goals that were set following the visioning exercise of 1991.

Despite these good intentions, however, it became clear early on that changes in the budgeting process could not be instituted until issues involving the delegation of authority and control over resources were addressed. In effect, the budget process should reflect the responsibility structure in the organization rather than dictating it. The commitment was made to change the responsibility structure such that it, and the resulting budgetary process, aligned with the organizational decision-making process.

The Functional Organization

Historically, in Canadian health care organizations, structures have been influenced by the funding mechanisms imposed on them by government. The global funding system was built around the idea that an organization should be given a block grant with which to perform all services required for the patient population. In order to determine the size of this block grant, operations were reviewed by the provincial Department of Health on a function-by-function basis. Determinations were made as to the amount of funds required to provide specified volumes of laboratory services, nursing care for the patient population seen by the organization, housekeeping services, utilities and maintenance services, transcription and dictation in medical records, administrative support sufficient for the size and complexity of the operation, and all the other functions associated with the operation. In effect, the global grant for the hospital became a number of subgrants associated with specific functions or specialties.

Organizing around these subgrants made some obvious sense since there would be a link to the government funding system. Each year the global grant would be increased by a flat percentage, which could then be applied to the functional areas in the same way. Expansion of and additions to programs and services could be accommodated within the functional specialty with whatever funding had been granted by the Department of Health. In essence, funding determined the strategic direction of the organization. If the Department of Health was prepared to fund a program or service, then the organization would undertake to offer it. The hospital took on a functional focus, which meant that often new developments or improvements that were put forward for new funding were based on the provider's desires rather than on the needs of the ultimate consumer, the patient. New diagnostic procedures, changes in surgical techniques, and developments of new medical subspecialties led to requests for funding from the Department of Health to support the new functional enhancement. Acquisition of these increased the size of the budget, enhanced technical capacity, and hence were sought in their own right.

The corporate structure was organized in a similar fashion. Divisions were assigned to vice presidents, and a portfolio of functional specialty departments or clinical discipline was attached to each. Attempts were made to group these departments and disciplines logically: respiratory services, laboratory, and radiology might be pulled together into a diagnostic services portfolio; nursing would be captured in another; administrative and support departments went elsewhere. This encouraged loyalty to the functional specialty and made interaction and coordination between functional areas difficult. To overcome these integration difficulties, a large group of coordinating committees had to be structured to ensure that all points of view were presented in discussing major patient issues. Without such liaison devices, program changes in one area could have dramatic and unanticipated effects in another.

With this functional organization structure in place, the allocation of budget dollars flowed naturally according to delegated organizational responsibility. Functional specialty departments were granted set budgets each year. These were increased (or decreased) in accordance with government grants plus any program adjustments related to new operational initiatives. A system of responsibility accounting was used to establish cost centers for management control. The focus within these cost centers was on the objects of expenditure for that area—for example, medical staff fees, management salaries, wages paid for relief staff, regular wages, stationery costs, medical and surgical supplies, consulting fees, and travel costs. Detailed breakdowns of costs within each department provided considerable information on the cost of labor, mix of staff, rates of pay, utilization of hours, specific supply items, contracted services, and perhaps some miscellaneous recoveries from outside the institution such as the sale of instructional manuals or consulting services when provided by the department on a cost recovery basis.

However, a number of factors were missing. The objects of expenditure for the department cost center did not reflect capital items such as furniture, equipment, or other items having a useful life extending beyond one year. Nor was there a clear understanding of the impact these departments had on other areas of the hospital from which they were demanding services. For example, a nursing area would have a clear definition of the costs of nursing and medical/surgical supplies, but the cost of diagnostic services that were being requested by that area was not specified. Similarly, the work of the housekeeping department in maintaining that care area would not be captured as part of the nursing area budgets.

In areas such as radiology, there were considerable capital costs for equipment. Record keeping of such information was done on a central basis and was not made part of the data provided to the Radiology Department to assess its relative productivity or "return on investment." As a result, there was a very limited understanding within the department of all the cost elements directly associated with departmental operation on a day-to-day basis. All areas were treated as classic cost centers without regard for any revenue-generating potential, profit maximization, or return on investment.

The basic rationale for this cost center approach was linked to the government funding system since there was really only one major source of revenue—namely, government grants. As a result, no revenues could be attached to specific areas. Hence, no profits could be determined or returns on investment calculated.

In the functional organization approach, it was appropriate to focus on cost centers. However, this limited the ability to measure the effectiveness of resource utilization by the functional specialty since the only focus was to "live within the budget." Since the budget process was incremental, from each department's perspective, the larger the base budget the better. This made it easier for the department to live within the budget, and, if a period of restraint was imposed, it would be easier to reduce from an inflated budget figure than from a limited one. Any inequities that created either inflated budgets or inadequate budgets were only exacerbated by the incrementalism in the budget process.

Another major criticism of a process associated with "living within the budget" was a perceived lack of accountability by some organizational members. The service demands of one department on another were used as a justification for increases in the budget. However, the demanding department was not required to explain and justify the utilization. For example, physicians' utilization of laboratory tests could continue to increase without any financial consequence. The laboratory was expected to provide these services in unlimited quantities. As volumes grew, the only recourse was to request of central administration an increase in budgetary allocation.

In this context, most budget discussions centered around why the budget had to be increased. The major justifications related to volume increases that were viewed to be uncontrollable by the service provider. Interestingly, discussions concerning growing volumes occurred between the functional department and central administration rather than between the service provider and the service user.

The functional specialties had been organized in terms of divisional portfolios reporting to vice presidents. Members of management felt a loyalty and obligation to their vice presidents, who in turn felt an obligation and commitment to obtain the necessary resources for their portfolio departments. Any discussions surrounding rationalization or mediation of allocation decisions had to take place at the senior management level. Resource allocation decisions made at that level would then be disseminated downward into the organization.

As a result, the organization structure promoted highly centralized decision making, and the resource allocation process was a direct reflection of that centralized approach. The information gaps at the senior management level had the potential to lead to inappropriate decisions, some of which had to be overturned at a later point. This scenario led to a perception of unfairness, deals under the table, political intrigue, and general unhappiness and discontent with the resource allocation process.

Although the senior management team worked well together, the feeling within the hospital as a whole was that a broader group of people needed to become involved in these resource allocation decisions. It was obvious that physicians in the clinical leadership positions of the various specialty areas had to become more involved in the decisions related to resource allocation since they had different insights into operations from those of the people at the senior management level. However, attempts made to bring them into the decision-making process did not produce the desired results. This occurred primarily because the organization's responsibility structure continued to funnel the input of the physicians in those clinical leadership positions through one member of the senior management team, the vice president responsible for medical affairs, rather than through the clinical areas. Additionally, there was no incentive to bring together service users and service providers since budget dollars were obtained ultimately from a member of the senior management group rather than through departmental cooperation. Unless this organizational dynamic could be changed, it seemed almost impossible to fundamentally alter the budget process that was viewed so unfavorably by the vast majority of members of the organization. Operating departments needed to feel a sense of dependence on their customers and suppliers for financial and budget performance rather than dependence on a vice president.

Interestingly, these characteristics were present for many years but the degree of unrest and discontent heightened as two things changed in the environment. Internally, the advent of total quality management and the focus on partnership, empowerment, and the patient gave the organization and its members new lenses through which to view the budget process. Through those lenses, it became clear that a functional orientation limited the ability to focus on patient needs. In addition, a highly centralized decision-making structure at the senior management level did not support the concept of empowerment of staff throughout the organization. And, the departmental structure did not create an environment of partnership but promoted professional rivalries and independence.

The second environmental factor that altered perceptions was the advent of new funding mechanisms from the Department of Health as resources became more and more limited. A new plan created a funding system on the basis of cost per patient. This meant that the costs of all services provided had to be tallied by patient to determine whether the organization was able to operate within the funding being provided by the government for that particular type of patient. As resources became more limited and funding levels dropped, it became increasingly important to understand the hospital operation on a patient-by-patient basis rather than by functional department.

Together, these two factors led to a major reorganization that altered the decision-making structure in the hospital and paved the way for a new budget process. The new organizational structure created opportunities for interaction between previously separate functional specialties and spawned a new mandate to measure effectiveness on a multidimensional basis. It was no longer sufficient "to live within the budget." Success had to be demonstrated in meeting targets established for increased productivity and increased quality of service while also meeting the volume demands for patient service. The ground was now ready to plant the seeds of a new budget process—an internal economy.

Decentralized Patient Services Model

As was described in Chapter Two, the infrastructure is a complex web of policies, processes, and systems supported by a management hierarchy. The organizational structure has a profound influence on the operation of the hospital by creating patterns of behavior that directly affect the way in which work is performed. Sometimes these patterns of work are inconsistent with staff "doing things right." This was the essence of the message given by the hospital's chief executive in June 1993 in a letter to staff advising them of a significant and visionary change in organizational structure (D. P. Schurman, letter to staff, June 14, 1993).

The organizational structure at the University of Alberta Hospital was revised with six major goals in mind: (1) organizing or clustering services around the patient, (2) creating and reinforcing natural relationships of people working together, (3) bringing senior management closer to daily activity, (4) decentralizing decision making, (5) enabling greater accountability and responsibility for resource utilization, and (6) reducing management costs. Although the organizational change was initiated within a short time frame, the revised structure was the result of evolution surrounding total quality management and the influence of the associated principles becoming a reality in the organization.

A decentralized structure had been a commitment in a four-year strategic plan for the hospital that was approved by the board in 1991. This intention was reiterated in a statement of principles and commitments by the senior executives several months prior to the change. Throughout the organizational transformation, staff input was also continually sought regarding ideas, suggestions, and constraints experienced as the improvement of processes was attempted.

The new organizational structure is best described as a decentralized patient services model. Three vice presidents were selected to head up three patient services teams: (1) surgery, obstetrics/gynecology, anesthesia, (2) medicine/emergency/long-term care; and (3) pediatrics/psychiatry. To the extent possible, all resources and staff directly associated with the relevant programs were assigned to the areas. In addition to the three patient services teams, portfolios of corporate support and corporate development services were created.

The resulting structure meant that personnel in all health care disciplines, including physicians, were accountable through a specific vice president. Disciplinary divisions and segregated service departments were eliminated, and staff were positioned to work collaboratively as teams focused on the needs of specific patient populations. The new structure paved the way for an internal economy.

The Internal Economy

A major shift in thinking had to occur with the new organizational structure in terms of what the budget process really signified. Previously, it had represented the appropriation to departments of a portion of the total revenue available to the hospital. Now, the budget was to be viewed as a strategic tool—a mechanism by which scarce resources could be allocated to ensure optimal output. That output was based on the needs of the consumer and the strategic direction of the organization.

Clearly, as government grants began to shrink, all services could not continue to be supported in the same fashion as before. Choices had to be made. These choices would be reflected in an informational budget rather than, as in the past, in a pro rata reduction applied to all areas of the organization. Previously, the amount of money/budget available had determined the operational plans to be implemented. Under the new organizational structure, the budget would become an informational tool to translate strategic goals into a financial expression of the current year's operating plans and tactics.

The *internal economy* is viewed as a mechanism through which scarce resources are allocated in accordance with the strategic priorities of the organization. The commitment was to create an internal economy that would move the hospital from centralized planning toward relationships between organizational units based on responsiveness to patient demand. Although this economy would be a closed system and the amount of resources limited to a set amount, the allocation of resources would be fluid enough to respond to the fluctuating demands placed on the various areas of the hospital according to the number and severity of cases handled during the year. Clearly, if a component of the organization was on a track to overspend its resources, adjustments would have to be made. But now those adjustments would be made on the basis of strategic priority rather than pro rata adjustments.

New accountabilities were created by assigning to an identifiable organizational unit all those resources controllable by that unit and needed to provide service to its customers. The laboratory sells services to patient care units. Housekeeping provides services to the laboratory. The operating room sells services to patient programs. In cases where services could be completely decentralized, staff and resources budgets were moved out of functional specialty departments into the departments requiring services. Imputed revenue was calculated for as many areas as possible. The patient service teams that had been created in the reorganization were allocated revenue based on their case mix and the funding provided from the government for those patients. The laboratory received "revenue" from the patient service team based on the volume of tests negotiated with and provided for the patient service areas. Overhead items that could not be attributed to specific areas were charged to all areas of the hospital on a proportionate basis.

Through this process, "surrogate" revenue, profit, and investment centers were created. The performance expectations of these accountability centers were geared to strategic priorities and patient needs as well as to the expectations set to meet volume targets, quality of service targets, and productivity targets as negotiated between organizational units.

The organizational divisions produce annual operating plans based on a strategy that is outlined for and approved by the board. A forecast of revenue and expense is created. This becomes an informational benchmark against which actual results are measured. It does not, however, represent the amount each area has available to spend. The amount available to spend is determined by what the division is able to earn from its internal and external customers, and the expenses are determined by the amount necessary to earn that revenue. To reflect this in the reporting mechanism of the hospital, a flexible budget was created to ensure that performance assessments were based on revenues earned rather than on a fixed allocation.

As decentralization proceeded, it became apparent that several factors required attention and development. First was the question of which services should be decentralized and which should remain centralized. Second, a focus on service agreements was required. Information availability was also an important consideration.

As the budgeting system was brought into alignment with the organizational structure, the development and reflection of strategic priorities became more meaningful, as did the necessity of accommodating capital expenditures in the process.

Lessons Learned

As implementation issues were encountered and addressed, several themes began to emerge as lessons and topics requiring consideration and resolution. These themes related to services to be decentralized, service agreements between areas, information technology, resource allocation as determined in the budgeting process, and capital expenditures.

What to Decentralize

One of the first major issues associated with the changed resource allocation process was determining the new decentralized unit, given the functional structure. Three patient service teams were created, based primarily on the physical location of clinical services within the hospital. These tended to be grouped around the third, fourth, and fifth floors of the building and hence were grouped into patient service teams accordingly. It was relatively simple to amalgamate the direct patient care costs associated with nursing services in these areas and assign them to the new patient service teams since this was primarily a reconfiguration of the former functionalized nursing division. The larger question around decentralization concerned the services that previously had been centralized but should now be physically and accountably related to the patient services teams. Three questions had to be answered: (1) Which services should be completely decentralized to patient services teams? (2) Which services should remain centralized in support departments? (3) Which services should continue to be provided on a centralized basis but be paid for on a decentralized basis by the user departments?

Areas that were dominated by individual service and a high proportion of human resource costs were more easily decentralized, especially in areas where they were directly related to the provision or support of care or services to the patient. In this category were services such as housekeeping, dietetics, respiratory technology support, rehabilitative services, and social services. There were other areas where decentralization was viewed as inappropriate, primarily because of the particular services provided. Examples of this would be human resources, information systems, finance, and physical plant, although it was recognized that there were certain parts of these areas that could be decentralized at some future date.

The redesign of work was also necessary if some of these areas were to be properly decentralized. Simply to take fifteen people and distribute five into each of three different patient service teams was not viewed as a constructive method of decentralization. The ultimate goal was to redefine work processes such that a function that was formerly provided by fifteen people could be provided by twelve and then assigned to the patient service teams. This would accomplish decentralized decision making and responsibility while attaining financial savings in the process of work redesign.

Some of these decentralization moves are still taking place in functional departments such as medical records, information systems, and finance. In these areas, work processes are being redefined.

The shift between centralized and decentralized functions is not absolute. The extent of decentralization may change as circumstances change and the environment is altered. Further shifting between a centralized and decentralized approach is quite possible if the organization continues to be responsive to its environment. As a result, the physical location and decentralization of some services will have to be reviewed periodically.

Two types of areas present a particular challenge in the decentralization of services: (1) areas that have a large investment in physical assets where it would be impractical to decentralize completely and (2) areas in which there is a particular corporate need to retain control over these functions on a centralized basis. Examples of the former might include complex radiologic procedures or an audiology service. Functions such as legal services, and finance, human resources, and information systems illustrate the latter.

To varying degrees, all of these areas can operate on a fee-for-service basis. The difficulty is how to go about setting the prices for the buying and selling of these services. Does the buying department have the option of going outside the organization, or is it restricted to the internal department, hence creating a captive audience? The implication for such captive audience situations is that the prices set will be monopoly prices and that this may suboptimize utilization of resources throughout the organization.

The philosophical stance taken was that organizational departments would not go outside the hospital for services and that internal departments would have to meet pricing standards established by benchmarking and by comparison to organizations outside the hospital—either private sector firms or other hospitals. In this way, the captive audience would have some assurance that the service providers were at least as efficient as comparable providers outside the organization.

Within this framework the major concerns of the user departments involved the volume side of the negotiation and the quality of services to be provided. Historically, this had been the area of difficulty. In the past, volumes had been uncontrolled, by either the user or the provider, and changes in volume had been dealt with by making adjustments in the provider department's budget. Now, through the negotiation process, users and providers had to understand and specify the volumes expected, the related service commitments, and the conditions of satisfaction as part of the new dynamic between organizational units.

A line-by-line analysis of responsibility for price and volume was made for a number of items throughout the organization (see Table 6.1). As can be seen in the table, the majority of user concern and influence involves the volume issue, while the major concern for the provider is the cost of providing the service. Even within the cost-of-service arena, many factors are beyond the control of the provider to the extent that labor components tend to be set through negotiated salary rates.

Table 6.1. University of Alberta Hospital New Budget Process

	Responsibility for Price and Volume	
Expense	*Price*	*Volume (utilization)*
Labor	Human Resources	Operating department
Benefits	Human Resources	Operating department
Medical and surgical supplies	Materiel management	Operating department
Other	Materiel management	Operating department
Drugs	Pharmacy	Patient service team
Laboratory services	Laboratory services	Patient service team
Diagnostic Imaging	Diagnostic Imaging	Patient service team
Nursing	Nursing	Patient service team
Controllable overhead	Overhead department	Operating departments Increase during phase-in
Noncontrollable overhead		Decrease during phase-in

Through the process of continually refining this analysis of the controllability of a particular line item of expenditure, it was possible to focus the attention of users and providers when negotiating a fee for service on the important issues of cost and quality of service rather than on items of little value that had tended to be the focus in the previous system.

Service Agreements

A key to the fee-for-service arrangement was the creation of *service agreements* between users and providers that documented in sufficient detail the quality, quantity, and price of service. An understanding of quality of service was crucial so that price and volume tradeoffs at the expense of quality would not be implemented without appropriate discussion and consultation. The concept of "conditions of satisfaction," as introduced in Chapter Four, was used in the negotiation of service agreements to create disciplined conversation around the important considerations in service provision. Clarity around these conditions of satisfaction was important not only for structuring the basis of the "business deal" but also for creating opportunities for conversation between organizational units that might never have taken place in the past. This concept was instrumental in creating the new environment in which interactions and linkages between service user and provider ultimately affect the patients.

An important principle that was incorporated into the discussion was customer satisfaction and the distinction between internal and external customers. There could well be a situation in which the service provider and the service user come to a conclusion based on the internal customer's (the service user) view of "value added" that is in direct opposition to the external customer's (the patient) assessment of added value. Effective service agreements must understand and incorporate the external customer's idea of value.

This understanding reinforced the need for a total quality management approach to comprehending external customer needs, assessing how well they were being met, and taking steps to improve satisfaction levels. By making this part of the service agreement, negotiation with a more consistent focus on the patient was created.

Information Technology

As mentioned before, the functional structure had been in place for many years. As a result, the information systems developed in the hospital were largely focused on a functional approach to data collection and analysis. Some preliminary steps had been taken to create patient-specific costing in response to new national guidelines for health care reporting. These became very important as the new government funding mechanism came into effect. Suddenly, there was urgency to create complete patient-specific costing in order to better understand how the organization was performing relative to the funding received. These preliminary costing methods were ultimately instrumental in providing the information capabilities to support the decentralized patient service teams and to develop charging mechanisms for those areas that required fee-for-service treatment.

However, the historical reporting structure had never accommodated a flexible budget and certainly did not incorporate techniques to deal with such concepts as fee-for-service arrangements, imputed revenue, or contribution margin analysis. As a result, a fast-track approach to the development of new information technology for the forecasting, reporting, and support of the decentralized decision-making structure was necessary.

Once a model had been developed for the type of reporting that would be necessary using flexible budgeting techniques and transfer pricing, developing the specifics was achieved through multiple iterations. As much as possible, existing technology was used, with new pieces added on a month-to-month basis. Affected departments moved into the development loop as issues and components affecting their areas were being developed. As further iterations of the model occurred, there was opportunity to revise and upgrade the approach to techniques and measurements. This iterative process is viewed as a continual one—probably a useful approach in the context of a rapidly changing environment. The world of static financial information systems and reporting packages is gone; the movement toward flexible information is the way of the future.

Resource Allocation

Historically, each year's budget has been an increment or a decrement to the previous year's allocation. To the extent that the hospital board set a "no deficit" policy, this meant that the budget grew or contracted to match the government grant and, to the extent that this could be attributed to specific programs, those programs' base budgets would change. To the extent that no specific areas were designated for change, then all gains or losses were shared essentially on a pro rata basis.

With the implementation of the new budget process, the board took an active role in identifying corporate priorities and allocated resources accordingly. The new process begins with a discussion at the senior management and board level to identify the strategic priorities for the organization. This sets the parameters for the "macro" allocation of resources to the three patient service teams and the corporate support and corporate development areas. In addition, multidimensional targets are set to guide performance management evaluation using criteria for quality of service, volume of service, and productivity targets.

Such discussions were not part of the old budget process. This new process requires new and different information, including analysis of demographic changes, consideration of the role of the institution and its linkage to other health care providers in the region, and the financial constraints exerted by shrinking provincial revenues. Although the task is a difficult one, it is productive in the sense that it forces all to challenge the status quo. This is rarely accomplished in an incremental budget process.

To assist in the strategic priority discussion, resource allocation criteria were developed through consultation with stakeholders throughout the organization. This was an attempt to identify the characteristics of programs and services that were most important for the organization to fulfill its role and mandate. Six primary resource allocation criteria were established: (1) fiscal responsibility, (2) recognition of excellence from peer programs, (3) conformity to core values, (4) leading-edge activity, (5) well-developed partnerships, and (6) clinical uniqueness. These criteria continue to be reviewed and modified as they are applied since the environment and circumstances faced by the organization are changing rapidly.

As the health care system and environment change, the role of the organization may also change. As a result, resource allocation criteria must be adaptable. However, given the importance of providing a strategic direction for resource allocation, this process of discussion and priority setting is becoming more and more important. For the budget to be truly an informational tool to help support the strategic initiatives of the organization, there must be clarity around the strategic direction for the organization.

Capital Expenditure

As previously noted, one of the weaknesses of the previous system was the omission of any assessment of the effectiveness and utilization of physical assets. Many departments of the organization did not have complete cost information available to them to determine their relative efficiency or effectiveness. For example, in the food services area, direct costs associated with labor and food costs were readily available and prices in the cafeteria and snack bars were set with these in mind. However, by excluding costs of depreciation, space maintenance, utilities, and so on, a degree of subsidization was in place for these "commercial" activities. The same situation existed in outpatient, pharmacy, and laundry and linen services.

With the advent of the decentralized model, the strictly commercial areas needed to pay their own way. As a result, depreciation and cost items for maintenance and support services were incorporated into the financial reports wherever possible. In many cases, this meant a dramatic change in the rates that were charged to users either on an internal or an external basis. However, it allowed the commercial organizations to begin accommodating needs for replacement of equipment and reduced the subsidization burden that some overhead departments had been forced to bear out of hospital operating grants that were supposed to be devoted to clinical activities.

A logical extension of this was the creation of asset and inventory evaluations for these enterprises such that they could be treated like an investment center. For the commercial areas, it is important to create a better understanding of effectiveness and to create a "level playing field" when those areas are in direct competition with the private sector.

For areas of the hospital accessing dietary, laundry, and pharmacy services, all-inclusive rates created a stronger appreciation of the cost of providing these services. One of the major criticisms of the former functional structure was the perception that many items were "free." As negotiations took place between laundry users and laundry providers, it became clear that these supplies and services were certainly not free and that cost included an extensive infrastructure that also had to be serviced.

Similar evaluations and understandings were created in areas such as laboratory medicine and radiology. This achieved a much better understanding about the necessity to fully utilize very expensive assets so as to reduce the unit cost to as low a level as possible.

The New Budgeting Process

With the decision to move to an organizational structure focused on the patient, new budget processes were crafted to support the new decision-making philosophy. Although many issues have been addressed, it is recognized that refinements will be necessary in the coming years as circumstances in the environment change or as the approach and philosophy in the organization are refined. This stance is viewed as both appropriate and beneficial so that, unlike in the past, the organization does not become comfortable with maintaining the status quo.

With a new decentralized decision-making focus, the organization's members are now more empowered with a budget process that encourages a focus on patient satisfaction. Decisions related to expenditures of resources have been moved into the areas that are most closely associated with providing patient care. Partnerships are now actively sought or encouraged through a negotiating process that requires service agreements between service users and providers.

Above all, strategic priorities focused on patient need have been enhanced by a process that begins with difficult discussions related to allocation of limited resources to meet multiple expectations about volume, quality, and efficiency of service provision in the patient service teams. In a total quality environment, the infrastructure now aligns with the context. As the budgeting process is continually improved, the manner in which other parts of the organization can address their quality issues is also enhanced and improved. This alignment of infrastructure with context within the organization becomes an important lever in enabling continuous improvement throughout.

Reference

Wildavski, A. *Budgeting—A Comprehensive Theory of Budget Process*. Boston: Little, Brown, 1975.

Chapter Seven

Measurable/Observable Results: Understanding Clinical Variability

Ronald H. Wensel

The power of total quality management as it is applied to clinical care and services is inherent in the principle of measurable and observable results. Through the understanding of processes and the measurement of specific variables relative to clinical activity, the identification of unexplained variations can provide important information about how to improve patient care. Scrutiny of specific variables, the reasons for differences in practice patterns, and the degree of agreement of desired courses of action intended to improve care are all part of the measurement and observation of clinical variability.

Consider the following examples of variability. According to the principal report of the Conseil d'Evaluation des Technologies de la Santé du Québec (1993), there was statistically significant variation in rate (that is, the number of times a procedure was performed per 10,000 people) between regions within the Province of Québec, within Canada, and between countries for such procedures as tonsillectomy, coronary artery bypass, cholecystectomy, herniorrhaphy, prostatectomy, hysterectomy, and appendectomy. A recent report by Every and others (1993), noted that the rates of cardiac catheterization after acute myocardial infarction varied significantly between hospitals with and without on-site cardiac catheterization facilities. Yet admission to hospitals with these facilities was not associated with improved short-term mortality rates.

Even within the same hospital, physician practices may vary remarkably. For example, James (1993) reported wide variation among sixteen urologic surgeons with respect to the length of time spent and the number of grams of prostatic tissue removed when performing transurethral prostatectomy. Paradoxically, the amount of prostatic tissue removed was inversely proportional to the surgeon's procedure time. On average, the shorter the procedure time, the greater the amount of tissue resected.

The principal benefit of measuring variation is to identify opportunities to improve. Consider the following (Berwick, 1991, p. 1218): "Why is the understanding and control of variation so central to improving quality? The answer, simply put, is that variation is a thief. It robs from processes, products, and services the qualities that they are intended to have." Berwick suggests that, in the assessment of variation, it is important to determine where it exists, whether it is desirable or undesirable, its cost, and its causes. This will lead to an understanding of how variation can best be reduced.

Historical Perspective

Although the impetus for measuring variability as a means to identify opportunities to improve has been attributed to Shewhart (1931, 1939), Deming (1986), Juran (1988), and others, the essence of the principle in the practice of medicine can be traced as far back as the seventeenth century. According to White (1993, p. 12), Petty (1623–1687), in his classic volume *Political Arithmetick* (1690), challenged his British colleagues in the Royal College of Physicians: "Whether of 1000 patients to the best physicians, aged of any decad, there do not dye as many as out of the inhabitants of places where there dwell no physicians." And, "Whether of 100 sick of acute diseases who use physicians, as many dye in misery, as where no art is used, or only chance."

White also reports that the "numerical method" as described in France by Louis (1782–1872) was the first attempt to apply statistical techniques in the assessment of clinical efficacy. Louis demonstrated that bloodletting, common in his time, was not beneficial and often harmful. He also challenged the concept that the experience of an individual physician was a reliable guide in the assessment of patients and that, to understand the origins, prevention, and treatment of disease, it was necessary to study large numbers of patients.

Florence Nightingale (1823–1910) is also considered by White to be one of the early pioneers of the uses of statistical methods in the assessment of outcomes. She is credited with describing the first uniform hospital discharge data set, in which she correlated mortality rates and functional restoration with diagnoses and treatments.

In the early 1900s, Codman ([1916] 1992), a Boston surgeon, attempted to introduce a system he described as the "End Result Idea" for measuring outcomes at Massachusetts General Hospital. The essence of his system was that "every hospital should follow every patient it treats long enough to determine whether or not the treatment was successful, and to inquire if not, why not, with a view to preventing similar failures in the future" (p. 3). To this end he introduced a coding system to classify the causes of poor results according to errors in skill, judgment, lack of equipment, the patient's unconquerable disease, or refusal of treatment. Unfortunately, he was not understood and was forced to leave the institution. However, he did not give up on his concept; later he became a founding member of the American College of Surgeons and chairman of its first Committee on Standardization of Hospitals.

Another milestone portrayed by White pertains to Glover, an English physician who, in 1938, described wide variations in tonsillectomy rates among different surgeons and in different communities. Prompted by this "Glover Phenomenon" and other observations, White himself developed a population-based hospital discharge abstract system that was first implemented in Vermont. Subsequently, John Wennberg, a former graduate student of White's, has become an international authority in small-area variations.

Another former student of White's, Robert Brook (1973), together with Appel, compared five methods of peer review assessment of quality of care in terms of both process and outcome. Although the past quality assessment had emphasized medical process, Brook and Appel (p. 1327) reported major differences "between methods using process data and those using outcome data."

Disciplined scientific methodology was brought into the field by Bradford Hill (1952) through the introduction of the randomized controlled clinical trial. This robust scientific tool has achieved its present wide use through the magic of randomization, the discipline of blinding, and rigorous statistical testing. The randomized controlled clinical trial is regarded as the gold standard method for testing efficacy of clinical interventions. However, other research designs, such as time series studies, large ecological correlations, and before-and-after studies with controls, although not as powerful as the randomized clinical trial, are able to reliably test hypotheses or to identify unexplained clinical variation. All methods are of value in health care outcomes and in process research or quality improvement initiatives.

Clinical Variation

It is widely accepted that the 1990s will be the decade in which the traditionally autonomous element in the health care system, namely physicians, will become more accountable. In assessing cost and benefits of health care, it has become increasingly important to measure variations in both process and outcomes—process in terms of the cost/benefit of clinical diagnostics and interventions; outcomes as defined by death, disability, residual disease (infection rates, readmission rates), psychological distress, and patient dissatisfaction. All of this measurement is vital to improving the effectiveness, efficiency, and appropriateness of care.

Clinical variation can be measured in several dimensions: inputs, processes, and outcomes. In terms of inputs, there is variation in physicians' decisions to embark on particular treatment regimens. There are large differences among countries and regions in the rates at which many operations are performed. As was mentioned earlier, Every and others (1993) identified differences in the likelihood of cardiac catheterization related to the availability of such facilities, with no significant evidence of a difference in outcomes for the patients. Phelps (1993) reports a 16 percent rate for inappropriate hysterectomy among five health maintenance organizations.

As well, there may be wide variation among physicians within the same practice group with respect to the process of treatment. For example, length of stay for the same types of patients and the use of diagnostic procedures may exhibit wide variation within a geographical area or even between large teaching hospitals in the same academic medical center. As described by the American Hospital Association (1991), Chassin demonstrated threefold differences in utilization for 67 of 123 procedures studied. Other examples of unexplained variation included differences among like physicians in hospitalization rates, number of office visits, drug use, and use of diagnostic tests.

Assessment of variation in outcomes presents even more of a challenge. Outcome, according to Brook and Appel (1973, p. 1323), refers to the results of care—"mortality, symptoms, ability to work or perform daily activities, and physiologic measurements." They report, however, that outcome indicators of vital importance to the patient—activity and symptom levels—do not correlate significantly with judgments about the quality of care.

Other confounding factors in the assessment of outcomes include referral bias, patient treatment preferences, financial incentives or disincentives, and the training and experience of individual surgeons.

The principal benefit of measuring variation is identifying opportunities to improve. It is widely accepted that physician practice patterns change when unexplained and inappropriate variation is identified. According to Greco and Eisenberg (1993), the greatest impact on physician practice occurs if the information relating to variation is handled in a nonpunitive manner.

Traditionally, clinical review or audit data were used to set minimum standards for physicians. Within the newer context of total quality management, feedback of physician-specific information is best offered confidentially and in an aggregate, nonthreatening form to practice groups without asking for explanations as to why variations exist. Often physicians do not know they are at variance with their peer group. Changes are more likely to occur in a supportive, nonthreatening environment and if data are understood and accurate. The likelihood of change when inappropriate variation is shown is greatest among physicians and other health care professionals who take professional pride in providing the best possible care and who are committed to acting on behalf of and in the best interests of patients.

Measuring Variation

Approaches to measuring variation may be prospective, concurrent, or retrospective. Randomized controlled clinical trials exemplify a prospective method of introducing a manipulated variable—a particular intervention—using scientific methods including random assignment and blinding of subjects. Many drug trials fall into this category. The variation and effects are assessed before the results of the intervention are made generally available to patients.

An example of a concurrent method of variability measurement is occurrence screening against quality indicators determined by consensus of caregivers, as first described by Craddick (1979). A detailed description of this method is provided later in this chapter.

Retrospective variability measurement is illustrated by traditional quality assurance activities—medical chart reviews for morbidity, mortality, utilization management, medical record completeness, and blood product usage.

The overall goal in measuring variability, according to the American Hospital Association (1991, p. 7) is

> to provide physicians and other caregivers with meaningful information to support optimal clinical decision making and evaluation. . . . Valid and reliable information empowers sound decision making and ensures effective management, with the ultimate goal of improving the quality of patient care. In addition to the different approaches identified above, there are different methods to measure variation in health care. Commonly, differences in length of stay and resource utilization are measured using Diagnostic Related Groups (DRGs) in the United States or Case Mix Groups (CMGs) in Canada. This information, which may be adjusted for severity using Resource Intensity Weights (RIWs), Resource Grouper Numbers (RGNs), or one of numerous commercial systems, is particularly useful in physician practice analysis within hospital settings.

Clinical Practice Guidelines

Another method for measuring clinical variance and improving quality of care is described by Chassin (1993, p. 40) in his discussion of practice guidelines: "They represent the best synthesis of available clinical research and expert clinical judgment, created in an attempt to specify how health care should be delivered to minimize quality problems. Guidelines can be the template against which actual practice is measured to define areas of needed improvement." Practice guidelines are particularly useful in facilitating the assessment of appropriateness or inappropriateness in the use of specific medical services, such as nuclear magnetic scanning, or interventions, such as laparoscopic cholecystectomy. Measuring variance from clinical practice guidelines is one way to assess three varieties of quality problems described by Chassin (1993) as overuse, underuse, or misuse.

Clinical practice guidelines may lead into or merge with critical paths or algorithms, care maps, or decision trees. These appear to be most effective in reducing clinical variation if peer physician groups and other health care providers are involved in their development and implementation.

Population Health

From the broader perspective of population health, methods to measure variance are useful in assessing outcomes of care using such indicators as cholesterol levels, pap smears, breast screening, prostatic specific antigen screening, periodic health examinations, and management of hypertension. Ideally, determination of variation in outcomes should facilitate measurement of efficacy and effectiveness in the assessment of technology and performance. Unfortunately, the indicators of health status or outcomes of care are underdeveloped and are not yet uniformly reliable, clinically valid, specific, or widely used.

Models for Variability Assessment

Within the clinical practice environment in hospitals, the most successful approach to quality in terms of efficiency, efficacy, appropriateness, and resource utilization appears to be through the analysis of variance in physician practices. It should be noted that variances may be due to factors unrelated to physician practice. System process problems related to variation in physician practices typically involve factors such as inefficient support systems, inadequate communications, inaccurate data systems, outdated policies, and turf battles. Although much variation is unexplainable or unnecessary, some variation is appropriate and necessary to address patient-specific situations involving age, co-morbidity, or patient preference. The age, style of practice, training, and specialization of physicians may have a significant impact on their clinical choices and practice variations. Economic incentives and defensive medicine may also play a role in causing practice variances.

When selecting processes or clinical settings in which to measure variation, the greatest opportunity appears to exist where there are (1) high volumes of a particular diagnosis or treatment process, (2) high-risk procedures or conditions, (3) evidence of diagnostic and/or therapeutic variability, (4) sound scientific literature and comparative data, and (5) procedures that are likely to affect outcome.

At the University of Alberta Hospital, three interrelated programs have been implemented to measure quality of care and to identify opportunities to improve efficiency. Through measuring and comparing performance data related to caregiver practice (Clinical Quality Improvement), determining the clinical service utilization of resources (Patient Resource Consumption Profile), and comparing hospital resource usage profiles for specific cases to practice in other institutions (Value Improvement Process), significant improvements in quality of care and efficient use of resources have been realized.

Clinical Quality Improvement

The first program is a concurrent screening process known as *Clinical Quality Improvement*. In this program, objective quality indicators and criteria are used to review patient records in order to identify variations in medical and nursing care, processes, and outcomes. Screening also identifies problems with quality and/or variations in ancillary services such as respiratory, occupational, physiotherapy, and pharmacy services, as well as concerns relating to the infrastructure, such as environmental services and food and nutrition. Records are screened by analysts—experienced and specially trained nurses—at the time of admission, every forty-eight to seventy-two hours thereafter, and following discharge. Twenty-four generic criteria (indicators) that designate optimal practice in the various services and programs are customized to the service and agreed to by consensus of medical and nursing staff. Major indicators in the program are listed in Table 7.1. Each of these indicators or criteria has as many as ten subsets.

Integral to the occurrence screening process is the concept of continuously identifying variances, finding and removing the root causes, and measuring the outcomes and compliance to the action taken. Data and medical performance information, which are privileged under the provincial Evidence Act, are presented at monthly departmental and divisional meetings. The ensuing discussion focuses caregivers on assessment of contributors to the occurrences, actions surrounding the incidents and discussions concerning resource management to develop or change policies, procedures, or protocols. Action plans are developed, documented, and monitored.

Information is also provided for numerous quality management committees, including Infection Control, Utilization Review, Pharmacy and Therapeutics, Ancillary Support, Quality Appropriateness Review, and Mortality/Morbidity Review. The ability of each of these groups to use the data obtained by a single review enables resources to be used more effectively by preventing duplication of effort by analysts and committee members.

The Clinical Quality Improvement program is based on the premise that physicians and nurses, through education and discipline, are familiar with self-regulation and aspire to provide the highest-quality care possible for their patients. There is strong identification with the program amongst physicians, nurses, and

Table 7.1. Clinical Quality Improvement: Criteria for Assessment

Criterion 1	Admission for adverse results of outpatient management
Criterion 2	Readmission for complications or incomplete management of or problems related to previous hospitalization
Criterion 3	Operative/invasive procedure consent
Criterion 4	Unplanned removal, injury, or repair of organ or structure during surgery, invasive procedure, or vaginal delivery
Criterion 5	Unplanned return to operating room or other special procedure room on this admission
Criterion 6	Surgical and other invasive procedures that do not meet criteria for necessity and appropriateness
Criterion 7	Blood loss, excessive or inappropriate administration of blood/blood components
Criterion 8	Nosocomial infection (hospital acquired)
Criterion 9	Drug/antibiotic utilization that is unjustified, excessive, or inaccurate; that results in patient injury; or that is otherwise at variance with professional staff criteria
Criterion 10	Cardiac or respiratory arrest/low Apgar score
Criterion 11	Transfer from general care to special care unit
Criterion 12	Other patient complications
Criterion 13	Hospital-incurred patient incident
Criterion 14	Abnormal laboratory, X-ray, or other test results, or physical findings not addressed by physician
Criterion 15	Development of neurological deficit that was not present on admission
Criterion 16	Transfer to/from another acute care facility
Criterion 17	Death
Criterion 18	Subsequent visit to ER or OPD for complications or adverse results related to previous encounter
Criterion 19	Utilization variations according to medical staff criteria
Criterion 20	Medical record documentation deficiencies—physician
Criterion 21	Medical record documentation deficiencies—nursing
Criterion 22	Departmental or other problem(s)/ancillary department(s)
Criterion 23	Patient/family dissatisfaction
Criterion 24	Inappropriate discharge planning

paramedical departments and a sense of ownership that has resulted in commitment to quality improvement, consensus about process improvements, improved care of patients, reduced rework and duplication, and improved efficiency.

For example, at a regular meeting of the Division of Gastroenterology, process improvements were initiated in regard to (1) therapeutic levels of nephrotoxic antibiotics, (2) responsibility for follow-up orders after therapeutic intervention, and (3) resident teaching with respect to quality improvement orientation, adverse patient occurrences, and the involvement of residents in process improvement activities. At the University of Alberta Hospital, the identification of quality-of-care issues has proven to be an additional and effective method of enhancing clinical training for resident physicians. In this era, when economic realities are driving changes in health care paradigms, it is important that in the training of future graduates academic medicine reinforces the concepts of accountability and continuous quality improvement.

Patient Resource Consumption Profile

The second program, the *Patient Resource Consumption Profile*, focuses on resource utilization. It involves the regular presentation of aggregated data by case mix group, physician, service, or department. The objective of this review is to compare patterns of care and/or variations in treatment with the goal of using hospital resources in a cost-effective manner.

To provide this information, the University of Alberta Hospital has developed a specific costing system—the Patient Resource Consumption Profile (PRCP)—which measures exact costs for laboratory, radiology, nursing, rehabilitation, and operating room services. In the future other cost components, including medications, will be added into this computerized system. Length of stay and PRCP cost information is presented regularly in a blinded manner to peer groups of physicians or surgeons caring for patients of a similar case mix.

In this way, best practices are identified. Based on this information, in most instances, physician groups themselves have initiated changes in practice patterns that have resulted in reduced variation within peer groups, and also between hospitals, using data from comparable institutions. As a result of this program, noteworthy reductions in resource utilization have occurred in coronary artery bypass grafting, cholecystectomy, normal deliveries, cesarean sections, lens replacement, and transurethral prostatectomy. Along with other measures, this program has contributed to the overall reduction in length of stay for patients at the University of Alberta Hospital from slightly over 8 days in 1990 to 6.55 days in 1993. While the cost of care and length of stay have been reduced (as have total hospital expenditures), clinical volumes and quality of care, as assessed by concurrent screening in the Clinical Quality Improvement program, have been maintained or improved. In some programs, reductions in the length of stay and cost of care have been dramatic. Figure 7.1 illustrates a comparison of costs in two consecutive groups of open-heart surgery cases. For a larger number of patients, costs decreased in terms of laboratory tests, radiology examinations, operating room use, and nursing care. Length of stay decreased from an average of 3.3 to 2.2 days in the intensive care unit, 8.4 to 6.3 days on the postoperative ward, and 15.8 to 13.0 days for total hospitalization. Each of these changes was significant with p values less than 0.002.

Value Improvement Process

The third program to measure clinical variability is based on the *Value Improvement Process* introduced to the University of Alberta Hospital by the Baxter Corporation. Through this process, specific component costs of care for certain high-volume/high-cost procedures are identified. Components include the separate and specific costs of supplies (including prostheses), drugs and intravenous therapy, room and care (including nursing care), blood and related

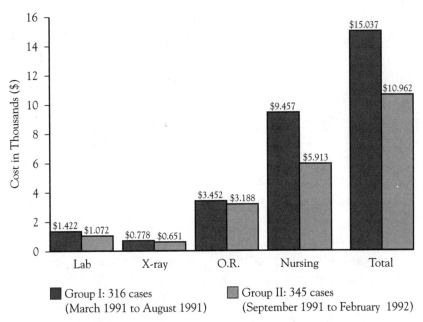

Figure 7.1. Cost Reductions for Open-Heart Surgery.

Source: University of Alberta Hospitals, Patient Resource
Consumption Profile Data, 1992.

therapy, laboratory services, and operating room costs. Each component cost is then compared with the best demonstrated costs in other benchmark institutions to determine the magnitude of opportunity for improvement.

As illustrated in Figure 7.2, the costs of the above-mentioned factors for total hip replacement were examined. By using the best demonstrated cost from all institutions as a basis for comparison, an opportunity for improvement was identified. In the case of total hip replacement, that opportunity was $2,330 per case (University of Alberta Hospitals, 1991). Through benchmarking with other organizations, the caregivers then determined how they could improve performance in the areas offering the greatest opportunity for improvement. By implementing these changes, significant cost savings were realized.

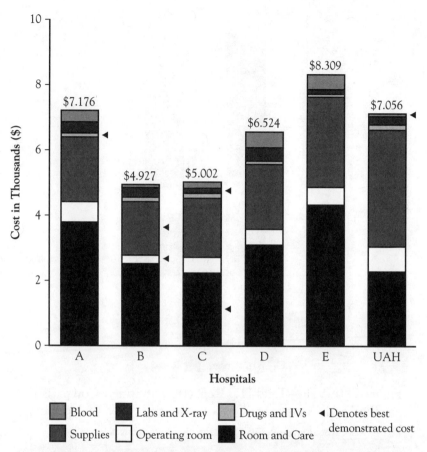

Figure 7.2. VIP—Total Hip Replacement Study: Comparison of Total and Component Costs Among Similar Hospitals.

Source: University of Alberta Hospitals, 1991, p. 3.

For total hip replacement, changes in costs for supplies, drugs and intravenous services, room and care, and laboratory tests resulted in a 21 percent reduction in total cost per patient, a 13 percent reduction in total expenditures on the nursing units, and a reduction in average length of stay from 8.6 to 7.5 days (University of Alberta Hospitals, 1991, p. i). The cost per case decreased to $5,563 from $7,056. Figure 7.3 illustrates these savings.

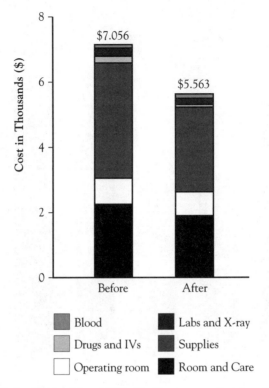

Figure 7.3. VIP—Total Hip Replacement Study: Comparison of Total and Component Costs Before and After Reductions.

Source: University of Alberta Hospitals, 1991, p. 9.

This program has resulted in significant cost savings in hip replacements, abdominal cholecystectomies (although laparoscopic cholecystectomy has changed that picture), full-term normal deliveries, and coronary artery bypass grafts.

Critical Success Factors

The American Hospital Association (1991) has identified five basic elements for success that must be attended to when implementing programs such as those described above.

Physician Leader Involvement

There must be support, advocacy, and active participation on the part of physician leaders within the institution. At the University of Alberta Hospital, the Vice President (Medical Affairs), the president of the medical staff, and the chairman of the medical staff advisory board (Medical Advisory Committee) were instrumental in and supportive of the development and implementation of the program. The Vice President (Medical Affairs) became the champion of the programs and, in the broader sense, of the organizational commitment to total quality management. The president of the medical staff (who was also surgeon-in-chief of orthopedics) became one of the first practitioners to become involved in all three programs.

Goal Clarification

It is important to clarify for the practitioners participating in them the goals and uses of the programs. Of utmost importance is the emphasis on improvement of patient care—an element that is of vital concern to the professionals providing that care.The programs are not intended to single out underperformance or to only reduce cost.

Management of Data

Careful management and communication of data is stressed by the American Hospital Association (1991). Information should be presented in a nonpunitive, nonthreatening manner to peer groups. It is equally important to ensure that the data are accurate and are presented in a format that is easily understood and meaningful. While particular data should not be published, they must be made available to peer groups if staff are to become engaged in the identification of inappropriate variation and the changes necessary for quality improvement. If managed in this way, reliable data become the driving force for change and health care providers can be expected to make informed clinical judgments that improve quality of care and, at the same time, reduce the cost of care.

Institutional Support

There must be institutional support for programs such as those described above from the technical perspective of data collection and analysis. The administrative reporting structure may play an important role in the promotion of physician confidence in the system. For instance, to obtain trust and dispel the notion that quality improvement initiatives could be threatening to individual physicians, in the beginning it may be necessary to develop programs and supporting data bases that are within the sole jurisdiction of physicians.

Communication, Patience, and Perseverance

In any institution or organization, change may be threatening, especially if individuals do not understand, or are not fully informed of, the context in which change is occurring. The economic imperative to provide the best care at the best cost with a minimum of unexplained, inappropriate variation is just beginning to surface in the consciousness of many physicians. As this represents a historic change from generally autonomous physician practices to an era of increasing accountability, it is important that the introduction of programs be incremental, open, and transparent so as to obtain increasing involvement, commitment, understanding, and acceptance on the part of the entire team of health care providers.

Lessons Learned

Obviously, the exploration of critical success factors presented in this chapter points to a number of lessons with respect to successful implementation of programs focused on the assessment and measurement of clinical variability. Attention to these will certainly pave the way for success in the achievement of observable and measurable results as quality improvement is sought in patient care.

The health care system is fertile ground for quality management. Its professional groups generally have advanced educational preparation, a commitment to providing the best care at the best cost, professional pride to do the best they can for patients, and the historical background of improvements based on scientific measurement.

If physicians are given accurate data about inappropriate or unexplained variation in a nonthreatening manner, their practice patterns will change over time. Physician performance is more likely to change if practice data reflect aggregate, individually blinded information regarding processes or procedures.

The transition from autonomous physician behavior to accountability for outcomes and resource utilization represents a transformation that can occur only over considerable time—a journey of as many as five to seven years—and only if nurtured by administrative and physician leaders with the management philosophy, commitment, energy, and communication skills evidenced in an environment committed to total quality management. At best estimate, among medical staff at the University of Alberta Hospital, only about one-quarter of the quality journey has been completed. To facilitate this journey, extensive training programs have been developed for front-line workers, management, medical staff, and other health professionals in regard to group action, working together, facilitating successful meetings, quality improvement tools, personal communication, and the principles of quality management. One of the most popular initiatives is the regular presentation of two-day workshops attended by physicians, nurses, and supporting staff who daily work together in collaborative clinical settings.

Eventual success, as determined by previously unheard of improvements in institutional performance, may only be possible with uncommon commitment of all health care providers to the mission, vision, and values of the institution. As suggested by Blumenthal and Meyer (1993), intellectual leadership of this transformation should be the responsibility of academic health care centers that, in the future, will need to become as adept in health services, process improvement, and outcomes research as they have been in biomedical investigation.

It has been suggested that much efficiency and improvement would result in the health care system if it were possible to gain control of unexplained clinical variation. As Berwick (1991) claims, variability is a thief. It results in wasted energy, loss of information, and confounding of variables truly affecting the outcome of health care intervention.

At the University of Alberta Hospital, the incremental introduction of performance information and the emphasis on quality management represents an attempt to arrest the thief. Through the use of data as a means to prompt discussion of optimal practice, clinicians, upon observing the initial success of early implementers, have begun to request inclusion in the programs at the earliest possible date. The understanding of the importance of measuring and observing the process and outcomes of clinical practice is increasing in the minds of many—and may prove to be the key to continued viability of the health care system.

References

American Hospital Association. *Practice Pattern Analysis: A Tool for Continuous Improvement of Patient Care Quality.* Chicago: American Hospital Association, 1991.

Berwick, D. M. "Controlling Variation in Health Care: A Consultation from Walter Shewhart." *Medical Care,* 1991, 29(12), 1212–1225.

Blumenthal, D., and Meyer, G. S. "The Future of the Academic Medical Center Under Health Care Reform." *New England Journal of Medicine,* 1993, 329(24), 1812–1814.

Bradford Hill, A. "The Clinical Trial." *New England Journal of Medicine,* 1952, 247(4), 113–119.

Brook, R. H., and Appel, F. A. "Quality-of-care Assessment: Choosing a Method for Peer Review." *New England Journal of Medicine,* 1973, 288(25), 1323–1329.

Chassin, M. R. "Improving Quality of Care with Practice Guidelines." *Frontiers of Health Services Management*, 1993, *10*(1), 40–44.

Codman, E. A. *A Study in Hospital Efficiency*. New York: The Classics of Medicine Library, 1992. (Originally published 1916.)

Conseil d'Évaluation des Technologies de la Santé du Québec. *Variations in the Frequency of Surgical Procedures by Region in the Province of Quebec. (1) Principal Report. (2) Technical Report*. Montréal: Conseil d'Évaluation des Technologies de la Santé du Québec, 1993.

Craddick, J. W. "The Medical Management Analysis System: A Professional Liability Warning Mechanism." *Quality Review Bulletin*, 1979, *4*, 2–8.

Deming, W. E. *Out of the Crisis*. Cambridge, Mass.: MIT Center Applied Engineering Studies, 1986.

Every, and others. "The Association Between On-site Cardiac Catheterization Facilities and the Use of Coronary Angiography After Acute Myocardial Infarction." *New England Journal of Medicine*, 1993, *329*(8), 546–551.

Greco, P. J., and Eisenberg, J. M. "Changing Physicians' Practices." *The New England Journal of Medicine*, 1993, *329*(17), 1271–1274.

James, B. C. "Implementing Practice Guidelines through Clinical Quality Improvement." *Frontiers of Health Services Management*, 1993, *10*(1), 3–37.

Juran, J. M., and Gryna, F. M. (eds.). *Juran's Quality Control Handbook*, 4th ed. New York: McGraw-Hill, 1988.

Phelps, C. E. "The Methodologic Foundations of Studies of the Appropriateness of Medical Care." *New England Journal of Medicine*, 1993, *329*(17), 1241–1245.

Shewhart, W. A. *Economic Control of Quality of Manufactured Product*. New York: Van Nostrand, 1931.

Shewhart, W. A. *Statistical Method from the Viewpoint of Quality Control*. Washington, D.C.: Department of Agriculture, 1939.

University of Alberta Hospitals. Total Hip Replacement—VIP Orthopedics Study. Edmonton: University of Alberta Hospitals, 1991.

White, K. L. "Health Care Research: Old Wine in New Bottles." *Pharos*, Summer 1993, 12–16.

Chapter Eight

Process Management: Aligning Performance Competencies and Rewards

Lynn Cook

In the last chapter, the focus was on measurable, observable results, specifically as this concept relates to clinical practice. One of the "truisms" of total quality management is that "those results or outcomes that get measured (or observed) get managed." This is true not only for clinical care but for all aspects within a total quality management environment. In that regard, it applies to staff performance as well.

To illustrate this truism, consider a World Series baseball team. If the performance of the shortstop is based on how far the ball can be thrown, the player's attention and capability development will be directed toward throwing the ball greater and greater distances. But, what if, by throwing the ball as far as possible, it goes over the head of the player on first base and there is a failure to "make an out"? Surely the measure is on the "out" and not on the the distance. If that is the case, the focus for performance and performance improvement is on doing whatever it takes to make the "out," whether it is a long throw or a short throw.

If the organization focuses attention on one particular aspect of performance, staff attention will also be directed toward that aspect. The corollary is that, if an organization wants individual and collective attention focused on specific behaviors and results, then making available selective measurements will cause the attention

139

to be on those behaviors and results. The individual will be successful and, collectively, overall performance will lead the organization to achieve the desired transformation.

Managing performance within an academic medical center is a huge challenge. First, there is the sheer size of the organization, with large numbers of staff working around the clock each day of the year. In addition to size, there are complexities of varying roles; differing relationships between staff members, physicians, and the organization; as well as age, culture, education, and training. Finally, the rewards and recognition that are possible, or desirable, are not the same throughout. All of these factors dictate that performance planning, coaching, assessment, reward, and recognition be managed through a comprehensive, coordinated, and aligned system.

The development of a highly effective performance management system is essential. Excellent results can be achieved only though individual performance—performance that is focused on desired results, continually improved through capability development, and reinforced through appropriate rewards and recognition.

The principle of *process management* as described in Chapter Three was developed on this increasing understanding that the creation of a different future or improved results involves changing organizational processes and practices. Performance management serves as an example of how process management must be attended to if organizational transformation is to be achieved. In this chapter, the performance management system for the management staff at the University of Alberta Hospital is described. The group affected by this system is predominantly management personnel but also includes a small number of other staff not included in unionized agreements. In this chapter, the affected group will be referred to as the "management staff."

Focusing Process Improvement Efforts

As the University of Alberta Hospital's total quality management philosophy and strategy were rolled out within the organization, the need to focus individuals' job activities and expected results in a very different way became apparent. Changes included moving management activities from directing and controlling to visioning and planning, from acquiring budgetary resources to optimizing resource utilization, and from managing staff to leading and coaching. Several mechanisms aimed at shifting the focus were instituted. The new expectations were discussed throughout the organization. People were exhorted to change their behavior. However, the hospital's traditional performance appraisal approach continued to measure old parameters. These measures did not lead to a focus on the principles that had been identified as part of the hospital's total quality management philosophy or on the key results necessary to achieve the vision.

The management group expressed other dissatisfactions with the system. People did not know what was expected of them, and there were perceived and real differences in expectations for people working in various areas within the hospital. Rewards were still directed at the old measures—budgetary performance, individual relationships, volume of activities, numbers of reporting subordinates. Not only were the rewards inconsistent with the newly defined performance expectations but they were also applied inconsistently throughout the organization. It became clear that the lack of an effective way to manage performance was preventing a breakthrough in the level of individual and collective performance of the management group.

Given the strategic importance of an effective performance management system and the obvious problems with current practice, consideration was given to interventions that would improve the chances of making a positive difference. Assessment of current practice in light of the hospital's Organization Capability Development Framework described in Chapter Two resulted in a thorough review of the aspects of potential nonalignment—both among components and with other parts of the organization's initiatives—within the domains of context, infrastructure, and member capability.

Context

As a first step, the elements of the *context* within which leadership performance was planned, implemented, and assessed were considered. Both the hospital's mission and vision clearly articulated the key roles played by staff in the future success of the organization. The values of respect, partnership, and continuous improvement also pointed to behaviors and attitudes that are expected. It was evident that there needed to be a change in the performance management system if it was to align with the organization's new context. This new system would also be key in attracting, retaining, and empowering a team of highly capable individuals to design and manage the organization.

Infrastructure

Second, the assessment focused on the *infrastructure*—the systems, processes, and procedures in place to support performance management. Here there were some serious gaps. The way positions were defined had not been updated to reflect the total quality management environment and approach. Job description documents still defined management roles in terms of traditional direct-and-control activities and job scope related to budgets, number of employees, and reporting hierarchy. The factors used to establish the relative value of management positions had not been reviewed for many years; they reflected an organizational design from the past that emphasized individual performance, not team performance.

The existing performance-planning process directed attention toward tasks and was inadequate as a mechanism to promote and encourage competence surrounding expected behaviors or breakthrough results. Consequently, it was infrequently used and, when applied, did not provide an energizing and empowering conversation around performance and capability development.

In addition to outdated performance appraisal methods, the compensation administration system was poorly defined, particularly as it related to reward and recognition for excellent performance. It was also inconsistently applied. Clearly, there was a need for a major overhaul of the infrastructure surrounding this key strategic business process of performance management.

Member Capability

The third and final part of the review related to *member capability*, which includes knowledge, skills, and commitment. In the past, performance planning had been based on activities, not outcomes. Therefore capability gaps existed in (1) defining key results in a way that makes a difference for the customer and (2) measuring progress. Another area requiring new learning was the articulation of specific behaviors—the "how" of the position—in a way that promotes individual growth and development. Coaching was a new skill to many, and its critical impact on managing and developing performance meant that training and education were needed. It was clear that opportunities for improvement existed in the component of member capability.

Redesigning the Performance Management System

From the information collected through review of the organization's context, infrastructure, and member capability, and discussions with the members of the management group, a major project was launched to redesign the performance management system. The redesign efforts were spearheaded by a design team but the process provided for wide involvement of those affected by the anticipated changes.

When the activities surrounding the redesign were initiated, the focus was on compensation since that had been an area of significant dissatisfaction among management personnel. Of course, a factor in this dissatisfaction was the perception of many that individuals were not being compensated "fairly" given their relative responsibilities and level of performance in the organization.

The Design Team

A team of people was selected from among the members of the management group affected by the performance management system. Members of this design team represented a broad cross section of the job categories and the functional and program areas distributed throughout the organization. The initial purpose of the design team was to coordinate the development of a management compensation system including plans for implementation and evaluation. The associated objectives were to (1) ensure input fully representative of all stakeholders, (2) become aware of state-of-the-art practices in management compensation, (3) consistently manage the process according to the total quality management principles, and (4) recommend a new management compensation system to the hospital's senior decision-making body.

To initiate this work, the design team considered comments that had been solicited from all members of the management group at a management retreat. Retreat participants had been asked to define the circumstances under which they would feel totally compensated. Three primary themes emerged: intrinsic rewards, job characteristics, and monetary rewards.

In describing the factors that would make them feel "truly compensated," retreat participants had described a number of intrinsic rewards. These tended to illustrate their feelings about their work and their jobs. Included were descriptors such as "happy," "fulfilled," "enjoy what I'm doing," and "a sense of pride and personal success."

In addition to intrinsic rewards, several had commented on job characteristics that they would view as compensation for their investments and efforts in their work. Freedom and trust, the chance to learn and grow on the job, the ability to participate, meaningful relationships, and the sense that they and their work were appreciated were characteristics valued as components of compensation and reward.

Last but not least were characteristics of a system of monetary compensation. Retreat participants had stated that the system must be perceived as fair and equitable, with rewards related to performance. They felt that recognition in a monetary fashion was important and that this might take the form of bonuses or a share in the fortunes of the organization.

At the same retreat, participants were also asked to identify the elements of an excellent management compensation system. They had determined that a key requirement was a system that is clear and easily understood. Participants felt that it was essential to have a philosophy of management compensation that demonstrates the leadership role of the organization and its management group. Clarity of roles and expectations was seen to be essential. Words such as *openness*, *fairness*, *creditability*, and *flexibility* identified other characteristics. Participants felt that compensation must be linked to performance and that their performance should be assessed by peers, customers, employees, and the supervisor. Competition within the marketplace was also identified as an issue in the assignment of levels of remuneration.

In addition to the input received at the management retreat, representatives of the design team went to stakeholders within their specific areas to seek perceptions about the current management compensation system. The input received was similar to that from the management retreat.

Development work began and a set of guiding principles was established. The design team then spent several meetings discussing possible configurations for a compensation system.

After several months of work, it became clear that the project was much bigger than originally anticipated. The design team realized that a system for compensation could not be designed in isolation from an overall performance management system. In reality, this had been evident in the comments from the management group at the retreat—many of the descriptors about feeling truly compensated had nothing to do with financial gains. This learning was reinforced through the design team's initial deliberations, which shifted continually from salary and benefits to performance.

This realization was accompanied by the recognition that expertise on state-of-the-art performance management systems was not available within the organization. A decision was made to retain a consulting firm to provide expert advice to the design team. It was essential for organizational acceptance of the new system that the design be a local creation; however, supplementary expertise from specialists was required. Subsequent to a search and selection process, appropriate outside assistance was retained and developmental work began in earnest.

The Design Process

Once the decision had been made to undertake the development and implementation of a complete performance management and compensation system, the performance management and development cycle illustrated in Figure 8.1 guided the deliberations of the committee. Initially, attention to expectations was required. Second, the process associated with monitoring and review based on the expectations would need to be designed. Then the consideration regarding compensation would be timely and relevant. Finally, continuous performance improvement opportunities would be identified.

As the design team's work evolved, three major initiatives became important: the development of competencies to guide behavior, the specification of the performance management process, and the compensation process.

Development of Competencies

Performance within the organization came to be understood as consisting of two components: the way people behave and the results they achieve. The first major portion of the design work centered around the *development of behavioral competencies* designed to help managers understand the desired actions and how these fit into the

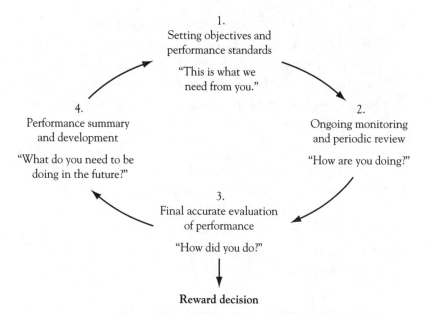

**Figure 8.1. The Performance Management
and Development Cycle.**

Source: Adapted from the Hay Group presentation at the meeting of the
Performance Management System Design Team, August 1992.

context of the organization. These competencies specified the
behaviors essential to the success of the individual in management
and, in turn, the success and transformation of the organization.

Using a predeveloped and pretested questionnaire, design team
members identified those behavioral competencies exhibited by
leaders in the organization who were truly successful. This list
became a working document for subsequent activities. From there,
focus groups and expert panels from the management group participated in validation of the identified competencies. The focus
groups validated the competencies by considering the successful
people in the organization and describing their behaviors. The consultant synthesized these behavioral examples into a description of
competencies. The expert panels then reviewed and ratified the
competencies. The result of this process was the definition of ten
essential behavioral competencies.

1. *Committed to the University of Alberta Hospital Vision*
   The ability to understand the goals of the organization and to align one's behavior with the vision. It involves acting in ways that promote the organizational vision or meet organizational needs, putting an organizational mission before one's own performance.

2. *Service Orientation*
   A desire to help or support others to meet their needs. It means focusing one's efforts on discovering how we ultimately meet customer needs. Customers are patients and their families, suppliers within or outside the hospital, the government, hospital staff, or any other person involved in health care delivery.

3. *Team Leadership*
   The ability to lead a team or other group. Also the capacity to create effective teamwork, either through direct action or by empowering team members.

4. *Decision Making*
   The capacity to select effective approaches to accomplishing tasks or solving problems while taking into account the needs and values of others.

5. *Resilience*
   The capacity to rise to difficult circumstances and respond in flexible ways while maintaining balance and composure. It also includes the ability to maintain stamina under continuing stress.

6. *Relationship Building*
   The ability to build or maintain congenial, warm relationships or networks with people that are aimed to be helpful in achieving work-related goals.

7. *Development Focus*
   The capacity to improve the performance of one's self and others through learning and development. This is apart

from participating in or sending others to formal training programs.

8. *Teamwork*

   The ability to work cooperatively with others as opposed to working separately or competitively. The team could be the formal work group or any other group of people functioning as a team.

9. *Achieving Consensus*

   The ability to reach consensus by understanding other people's points of view and adapting one's behavior. Also the ability to reach agreement in the face of obstacles.

10. *Innovation*

    The ability to improve individual or group performance by making comparisons, identifying patterns, and doing new things.

The descriptions of the behavioral competencies were important as a first step. However, in order to put these competencies into action in the performance management system, it was necessary to describe specifically the behaviors that would be demonstrated by individuals functioning at the various levels of competency. Thus, the behavioral competencies were further refined by the delineation of five levels of performance within each—from "not demonstrated" to "superior performance." Examples of each level were also articulated.

Table 8.1 lists the levels delineated for one behavioral competency—service orientation. The quotation associated with each level is an example of how individuals might illustrate the manner in which their actions reflect service orientation. For example, an employee who states, "Here is a copy of my letter of response to the patient who complained about having to wait for his test" is illustrating level 1 of service orientation. The person is following up on a complaint but not going beyond that to determine

Table 8.1. Levels of Performance: Behavioral Competence 2, Service Orientation

Service Orientation: A desire to help or support others to meet their needs. It means focusing one's efforts on discovering how we ultimately meet customer needs. Customers are patients and their families, suppliers within and outside the hospital, the government, hospital staff, and all others involved in health care delivery.

0   **Not shown:** This competency is not demonstrated.

1   **Follows up:** Follows through on customer inquiries, requests, complaints. Keeps parties up to date on progress.

"A patient who had been really unhappy with the service sent a letter. I personally called him to inquire about the incident and let him know what was being done to remedy the situation."

2   **Maintains clear communication:** Maintains clear communication with customers regarding mutual expectations. Monitors satisfaction. Distributes helpful information. Gives friendly, respectful service.

"I got the idea of having cards in every room asking for feedback about service. We now have cards in every room."

3   **Takes personal responsibility:** Takes personal responsibility for correcting and improving service. Acts promptly without being defensive. Makes self fully available, especially during critical periods. Takes extra steps to ensure personal availability to customers or may spend extra time servicing their needs.

"A patient was referred to my department by a physician for urgent care. The coordinator did not agree with the urgency of the request. I agreed with the physician and bypassed usual lines of authority to ensure the patient got the required care."

4   **Acts to make things better:** Takes proactive, concrete steps to improve the situation in some way. Expresses positive expectations about the situation and those involved.

"I set up an interdisciplinary committee to promote the use of infant safety restraints and develop a hospital-wide policy. We'd invested so much money in treating the effects of injuries, but not in preventing them. I wanted to change that. I think we really achieved something, and the really exciting thing about it is that the UAH has taken a leadership role within the province. It was a lot of work, but it's really important work."

Source: University of Alberta Hospitals Behavioral Competency Model, September 1992, Page 2.

whether long waiting times are usual or if something can be done to avoid them.

Again, review and refinement of the levels of competence were conducted with focus groups within the organization. The ten behavioral competencies and their levels of performance were then formally approved at a senior level within the hospital.

During the development of the behavioral competencies, extensive discussion occurred around the balance between behaviors and results. Results are described as specific outcomes associated with job accountabilities. They are expected to be concrete, measurable, and aligned with the strategic intent of the organization. For example, a key result associated with the behavioral competencies of the director of a patient service team may be that the hospital's mission, vision, values, and principles are reflected within the team. A measurable indicator of this would be the implementation within the area of a formalized strategic plan with obvious relevance to the hospital's strategic intent.

Is it acceptable for someone to behave in a superior fashion across all competencies yet not achieve results that truly make a difference for the organization? Conversely, is it appropriate for people to achieve key results while behaving in a way that is inconsistent with the expected competencies? The design team agreed that behavioral competencies and results were equally important. This position resulted in the development of a competency-based performance management system that includes planning and assessment of both competencies and results.

Performance Management Process

The next step in the work of the design team was to develop the *performance management process*. The objective of this work was to define a cycle that would reflect the four stages portrayed in Figure 8.1: (1) setting objectives and performance standards,

(2) ongoing monitoring and periodic review, (3) evaluation of performance leading to a reward/recognition decision, and (4) planning for the future.

In the development of the process itself, several objectives guided the work of the design team. The process was to be (1) meaningful, energizing, and enabling for those involved; (2) collaborative and ongoing with input from a variety of sources; and (3) an objective and documented basis for decisions about rewards and recognition based on both the "how" and the "what" of the job. It was also intended to provide a meaningful gauge for both the management person and the supervisor relative to the reflection of the organization's context, infrastructure, and member capability in the role performance of the individual and the team.

The resulting process is illustrated in Figure 8.2. Based on the ten behavioral competencies, the rater and the ratee together define the "how," identifying the level of performance required to meet job expectations and specifying examples of actions that would demonstrate the competency level identified. The second component involves defining job activities and key results, or the "what." This component forms a performance contract between the rater and the ratee.

Subsequently, there is a period of ongoing feedback and coaching as the role is being performed. Two interim reviews are conducted, plus an annual review to summarize the activities of the year and plan for the upcoming year. At this point, other raters identified by the ratee as individuals who have had an ongoing opportunity to observe performance of the behavioral competencies provide input to the review.

The complete cycle of performance management contributes to the integration of all aspects of the system: performance planning, development, career planning, succession planning, and rewards and recognition. This integration, in turn, leads to performance management system evaluation, adjustment based on that evaluation, and continuing process improvement.

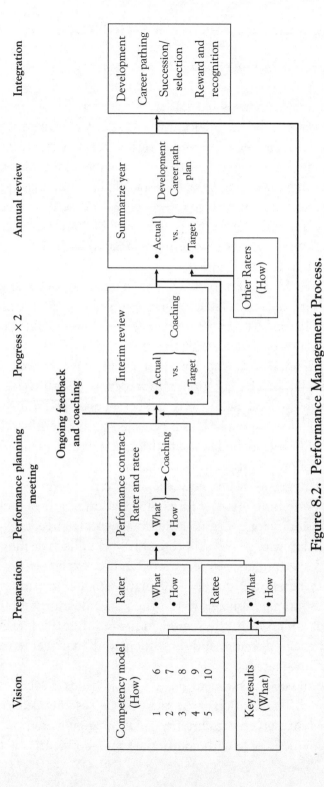

Figure 8.2. Performance Management Process.

Source: Adapted from the Hay Group presentation at the meeting of the Performance Management Design Team, October 1992.

153

Compensation Management

As the design team turned its attention to the matter of *compensation management*, the first major task was associated with the identification and classification of distinctive roles by the hospital's senior management to convey to staff the expectations associated with each organizational level in terms of accountability, output, activities, and capability. Five role levels were described, from the individual contributor to the fourth level of management—the chief executive. The specific terms associated with each of these roles are illustrated in Figure 8.3.

Just as each organizational level has a different role, so do various jobs within each level. Understanding these differences was important in establishing appropriate levels of remuneration.

The first step in identifying the distinct roles within the management group was to create a position evaluation questionnaire to analyze each job. The questionnaire was created within the management group. Role definitions had been developed using information from focus groups. This process led to the identification of factors that, when applied to the position description, distinguished the scope of one position from that of other positions within the management group. Six aspects of a position that were seen to differentiate one from another for compensation purposes included (1) responsibility for continuous improvement, (2) freedom to act, (3) overall knowledge and skill (breadth), (4) skills in dealing with people, (5) performance expectations, and (6) expertise (depth).

Thirty of approximately 150 management positions were selected as sample positions to test the job evaluation tool. Information obtained from the review indicated that the method of analysis appeared sound, and subsequently all management positions were evaluated.

Once all positions were evaluated, broad bands of salary ranges were created. The creation of the salary bands was intended to maximize flexibility, given the current, rapidly changing environment, and to provide people with additional job opportunities without significant concerns about salary changes. The objective when setting salary ranges was to ensure market competitiveness and internal equity.

Continuous Improvement

The final aspect of the performance management system is its ongoing management and *continuous improvement*. Just as the development of this system was spearheaded by a team made up of people affected by the system, its ongoing management will also be handled by a committee composed of members from the management group. The committee will be responsible for ensuring appropriate implementation, evaluation, and upgrading of the performance management system. Through rotation on and off the committee over time, all members of the management group will have the opportunity to become even more familiar with the management system and to contribute to its continuous improvement.

The initial urgency was to develop a performance management system for the management staff since it is these individuals who have the responsibility for designing and managing the organization. It is essential that the definition of roles and the clarification of expectations and rewards for performance are aligned with the total quality management environment. The performance management system is intended to accomplish that alignment. But a further question relates to applicability of this model to others within the organization.

Performance appraisal systems for other staff within the hospital have been revised and upgraded over time; however, the focus has been on the completion of forms rather than on the management of performance. It is intended that the concept and the approach used to develop the performance management system for the management personnel be applied over time throughout the organization for other groups, including unionized staff and physicians. There may even be applications at the level of the hospital board. Ultimately, the intent is to encompass the entire organization.

	Individual contributor	*First level*
Accountability	To perform, manage, and contribute to the improvement of the day-to-day work processes To contribute to the improvement of work processes on the work unit	To cause the implementation of work process improvements through: • Enabling the work group to continuously improve performance • Facilitating the enhancement of the capabilities of members
Output	Products and services that delight the customer	Well-running team (cohesive, effective, progressive, successful, happy) Cross-functional multidisciplinary problem resolution Optimal resource allocation and management Demonstrated improvement of work processes

Figure 8.3. Role Definitions.

Second level	*Third level*	*Fourth level*
To develop, integrate, and implement the mission/vision within the area of responsibility To lead to new levels of performance To champion departmental process through: • Defining the customers • Identifying customer expectations • Integrating work processes to meet and exceed customer expectations	To define and ensure implementation of strategic development To scan the environment To improve the health care system To create the organizational context To promote sustainable development (life) of the organization	Define the future Be a symbol (set the tone) Offer support (reason for action) Inspire (keeper of vision) Energize the organization Represent the organization Promote the organization Provide a systemwide vision of the health care system
Definition of departmental mission/vision and strategic plan Demonstrated improved performance as measured against customer expectations Demonstrated contribution to profession/community Quality indicators performance reviewed against indicators Cross-department collaboration	Definition of mission, vision and strategic plan Demonstrated improvement in organizational context elements Demonstrated contribution to the health care system Demonstrated improvement in major processes	Dynamic effective senior team Effective board Superior and improving performance of the organization Organization with sense of pride Shared mission, vision, and values

	Individual contributor	*First level*
Activities	Understand customer expectations Perform work processes Continually evaluate effectiveness of work in terms of customer expectations Identify, resolve, and prevent variances in work processes Work collaboratively to identify and implement work process improvements	Coaching Leading Facilitating Planning/scheduling
Capability	Competence in performance on the job Understanding of quality improvement processes and tools	Competence in performance of the job Coach Teach and facilitate Knowledge about budgets and enough information to make sound long-term decisions Knowledge of the capabilities of people on the team

Figure 8.3 (continued).

Second level	Third level	Fourth level
Optimize resource utilization	Develop corporate strategic and operating plans	Demonstrate unwavering commitment to the vision
Develop operational plans	Interpret the vision	Demonstrate systemwide thinking
Scan internal/external environment	Scan internal and external environments	Interpret and broaden environmental forces
Coach, lead, facilitate	Secure resources	Represent the vision internally and externally
Network and contribute to external community	Develop quality indicators and review against performance	Engage the board
	Network nationally	Coach, lead, facilitate
	Coach, lead, facilitate	Design a generative learning organization
		Create the context for achieving the vision
Value-added theory	Interpret the vision	Create and sustain the collective vision
Lead	Live the values	Ability in multidimensional thinking
Coach	Communicate	Ability to see and gain the desired future
Understand corporate process	Lead	Coach
Understand health care system	Coach	Lead
	Understand, interpret and apply quality improvement tools	Understand the societal and political context
	Understand health care system	
	Build teams	

Lessons Learned

The people in the hospital's management group indicated that change in the performance appraisal system was imperative. While the new system is in its infancy, informal feedback suggests that the new approach is a positive change. It is reportedly more objective than had previously been the case. It includes the opportunity for people other than an individual's supervisor to participate, which is seen to be essential, given the team approach of total quality management. It is believed that the use of this system will create consistency and alignment throughout the three domains that are vital to organizational transformation. There is confidence that, with the clearer expectations of individuals in their roles, there will be more clarity, certainty, and satisfaction in the process itself, resulting in effective use of performance-planning time and effort.

A key insight was the importance of both behavioral competencies and results to individual and, therefore, to organizational success. Early discussions within the design team led to the conclusion that they were equally important. At the time of publication, there was growing support for an approach that would see performance managed through the behavioral competencies with key results providing the focus for that performance.

It was important that the design process be visibly supported by senior officials in the organization. The executive team demonstrated commitment to this process from the beginning. Early in the development process, it was determined that the performance management system would be the basis for a somewhat expanded model to be used for performance management by the executive team. This expanded application reinforces the perception that the principles and general design parameters of the new system have corporate support. As the model was implemented, the president and vice presidents attended training sessions along with other affected staff members so that they would be fully prepared to participate as both raters and ratees.

The major issues associated with the new system arose during the implementation phase. The new performance management system affected approximately 150 management people. During the development, the design team, focus groups, and expert panels involved about 100 people. However, for many of them, involvement was fragmented, with participation in one piece of the project only. In addition, the major reorganization and downsizing as described in Chapter Six took place partway through the development and implementation. This resulted in changes in design team membership. The design team members therefore lost focus on the need and responsibility to communicate with the other stakeholders. As a result, when the model was completed and training was implemented, concern was expressed by a few of those less involved in the development about some of the fundamentals of the system. This was apparently due to their lack of ongoing inclusion in the evolution and development of the new system. However, once people had the opportunity to participate in the training programs, they felt more comfortable with the model and its potential. Nonetheless, the importance of ongoing communication during the design process to ensure acceptance was underscored.

Another challenge that arose related to time frames that were established for developing and implementing the training package and the performance management system itself. Incomplete training material that included a number of errors and inconsistencies added to the anxiety felt by the training participants. A more realistic time frame would have enabled the development of a complete and accurate training program and implementation schedule, which would have reduced the uncertainty and confusion of participants.

As mentioned earlier, major organizational changes occurring at the same time as the design work resulted in a number of management personnel leaving the organization and many others having their roles redefined. In this era of continual and rapid change, it was not possible to hold all variables constant while the transformation of another is occurring within the organization. However, a more deliberate assessment of the impact of a major change on other change initiatives might have led to the creation of opportunities for people to discuss emerging issues and to identify options for managing the interface among several key change initiatives occurring simultaneously.

The World Series champions introduced at the beginning of this chapter provide an example of how the top performance of individuals working together in a team can lead to excellent organizational results. As teams of health care workers strive for excellence, the organizational domains of context, infrastructure, and member capability must be in alignment to support this goal. As has been described, excellence in the delivery of health care is supported by an effective performance management process for all staff.

Reference

Hay Group. Adaptations from presentation materials used by consultants from the Hay Group during the development of the Performance Management System.

Chapter Nine

Customer Satisfaction: Redesigning Care Delivery

Heather A. Andrews

As the principles associated with total quality management became a reality within the University of Alberta Hospital, it became increasingly apparent that the business of care was structured to meet the needs of professionals within the system rather than the needs of the patients. The hierarchy was structured according to disciplinary functions; departments existed on the basis of historical origins rather than being focused on the processes of care. Staff performed their patient service roles from centralized departments and spent much of their time waiting to be called or waiting for their patients to be available for service.

With the introduction of total quality management, staff members became cognizant of inefficiencies and worked conscientiously to address them. However, it soon became evident that the "low-hanging fruit" in terms of reducing inefficiencies had already been picked and that ongoing changes in the system required a more pervasive and encompassing reform. The significant improvement in care processes and cost reduction that became necessary could only be realized through restructuring of the delivery of care and services to the patient.

This chapter describes initiatives undertaken at the hospital to redesign the systems of care delivery. While the full impact and outcomes of redesign cannot be measured as yet, the project is described to the extent possible at the time of writing. Readers interested in the outcomes of the project are encouraged to contact the University of Alberta Hospital.

Background

The University of Alberta Hospital was not exempt from the challenges facing health care systems in the early 1990s. Increasing demands; high costs of labor, technology, and supplies; quality issues; and progressive decreases in global budgets all posed a threat to the basic premises of the Canadian health care system and, in turn, the services offered by the hospital. Problems abounded, and these became increasingly apparent to patients, providers, staff, and government as fiscal challenges increased.

Early in the redesign process, an interdisciplinary group of physicians and staff began to define the situation from their perspectives. Problems clustered into five general categories: (1) personnel issues, (2) professional issues, (3) organizational issues, (4) resource issues, and (5) care process issues.

Personnel Issues

As was the experience of many other North American hospitals, the University of Alberta Hospital's proportionate allocation of the health care dollar became a concern. Lathrop's (1991) analysis of the health care wage dollar (see Figure 9.1), provides a pie-chart visual aid for examining the hospital's very similar pattern of resource use. An abundance of caregiver time within the hospital was devoted to documentation—much of which was never again consulted. The concept of structural idle time (waiting for action, time between tasks) was something to which everyone could relate. It was of great concern that such a small proportion of the operating resources was devoted to the care of patients.

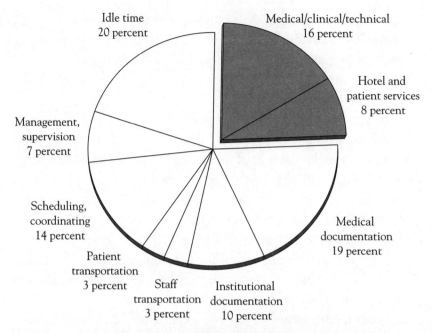

Figure 9.1. Breakdown of Hospital Employee Use of Time.
Source: Lathrop, 1991, p. 18, reprinted with permission.

There were many instances of inappropriate deployment of human resources, where people's capabilities were not appropriately matched with the tasks they were expected to perform. In addition, role confusion existed throughout the organization, and roles differed by time of day and day of the week. Staff felt that expectations were inappropriate, and, as a result, quality of care was compromised.

Professional Issues

Upon reflection, staff in the hospital began to understand that many of the problems being experienced were due to the locus of the processes in the health care system: serving the needs of the professionals rather than the needs of the patients. The entrepreneurial independence of a fee-for-service medical staff was manifest in a perceived unwillingness to change and reluctance to become involved in resolving problems of ineffectiveness and inefficiency. Interprofessional conflict was evident in attempts to protect "turf" and to withhold or manipulate information; this often took the form of subtle sabotage.

In nursing, the disciplinary evolution over the past several decades associated with professional credibility, educational preparation, and the delineation of a unique body of nursing knowledge accomplished much toward the professionalization of the discipline. However, in the effort to segregate a defined and independent role for nurses, barriers to interdisciplinary collaboration were erected. As described by Andrews and Wensel (1992, p. 29), "nurses as a category of health care providers gained a reputation for disinterest in interdisciplinary collaboration; they became perceived as more interested in protecting the role of the discipline."

Other health professionals also experienced conflict and insecurity. Discussion of cross-training, blurring of disciplinary boundaries, and the suggestion of "generic" health care workers who were not tied to specific units or specialties contributed to general suspicion, feelings of threat, insecurity, rigidity, and immobilization across professions and other types of work groups.

Organizational Issues

As the need for organizational restructuring and process redesign became more apparent, issues related to organizational behavior multiplied. Overlapping budgetary cutbacks and layoffs of staff contributed to uncertainty, fear, and a sense of impending doom within the hospital. It became apparent that further pro rata cuts in funding could be accommodated only by a drastic revision in the range of services offered; the mission of the University of Alberta Hospital as the principal teaching institution and tertiary/quaternary center would be adversely affected.

Although collaborative decision making and interdisciplinary problem solving were encouraged and supported, the traditional discipline-specific structure appeared to prohibit meaningful collaboration about the care processes. Support departments all functioned from a centralized base, and the prevailing understanding of processes and costs associated with any one clinical area was, at best, vague. There was evidence that staff were being stifled in their attempts to become involved in decision making—a symptom of too many managers and supervisors existing in the organizational structure.

Resource Issues

It was difficult to comprehend that a health care business existing in a spectacular physical facility such as that occupied by the University of Alberta Hospital could experience problems associated with configuration and technology. Nonetheless, problems did exist relative to both the allocation of technology and equipment and the layout of the physical space.

The Walter C. Mackenzie Health Sciences Centre at the University of Alberta Hospital was constructed in a time of great economic wealth in the province of Alberta. Its shopping mall atmosphere with two great central courtyards continues to draw the admiration of those who visit the facility. However, behind the impressive architecture existed problems related to the expense associated with upkeep and renovation and the proximity of services, as well as the challenges associated with staffing and managing small care units of eighteen beds.

Staff continually complained about the unavailability of such equipment as infusion pumps, and they perceived that technology to lighten their workloads was provided only in the intensive care units. Others observed that "high-tech" equipment was routinely used without consideration of what would be in the best interest of the patient. The status of information technology within the hospital and the adequacy of information required for decision making were also a concern.

Care Process Issues

Issues related to the care of patients abounded. From the perspective of staff members, there was a lack of understanding regarding the processes of inpatient care. The focus of most activity was on illness, with little consideration given to the patient's health status and need for care before and after hospitalization. Too often, care was perceived by patients as being impersonal, centered on technology and science, lacking in compassion, and often ritualistic; opportunities for education of patients and family involvement were often not pursued.

Although, through total quality management efforts, many staff and physicians were attempting to change care processes, the improvement activities were not coordinated. Initiatives were often duplicated, had effects on other areas, or were tied in to other interrelated processes.

These issues reflected many of the quality failures that Berwick and Plsek (1992) describe as being chronically present in health care: waste, inspection, rework, unnecessary complexity, defects, duplication of efforts, unreliability, letting people down, and making up to people for things gone wrong. All of these problems pointed to a need for significant organizational and process restructuring in order to accomplish the changes that would generate improved care of patients while accommodating cost reductions. As Curran (1991, p. 296) states,

> We've all been through budget cuts and every kind of budget-cutting process imaginable. We've all "tinkered" with approaches to decreasing costs and increasing productivity. Many institutions are into their third or fourth such cycle. Sooner or later all the "fat" is

trimmed and the budget arranged and rearranged every which way. Eventually, it becomes clear that we need to stop the tinkering and drastically change the way we do business.

Three years into the process of total quality management, it became clear that pervasive restructuring as addressed by Curran (1991) was required within the University of Alberta Hospital. The decision was made to embark on the journey of reengineering. The continuous improvement of existing processes was insufficient to address the need; the commitment was made to "start over."

Laying the Foundation for Change

The goals associated with the project of redesign from the organizational and patient care perspectives related to the problems that plagued the hospital. A primary objective focused on aligning the infrastructure of the organization with the context that had been created with the commitment to total quality management. As was described in Chapter Two, all aspects of the organization—context, infrastructure, and member capability—must be aligned if the organization is to respond effectively to the challenges facing health care and society in the 1990s.

The direction of the required change became apparent as the nature of the problems was analyzed: the organizational infrastructure must be designed around the patient. Only through this restructuring would it be possible to achieve the significant and pervasive changes required to improve organizational and care outcomes. Principles foundational to the organizational restructuring were those associated with the hospital's implementation of total quality management: effective relationships, empowerment and decentralization, accountability and teamwork, measurable/observable results, process management, customer satisfaction, and collaboration with partners.

The restructuring of the organizational hierarchy, as presented in Chapter Six, set the stage for the reengineering of patient care processes as described in this chapter. The objectives of this restructuring included (1) the organization of services around the patient, (2) the creation of natural working relationships, (3) moving senior management closer to the daily activities associated with patient care, (4) the decentralization of decision making, (5) the alignment of accountability for expenditures and, last but not least, (6) cost reduction.

The Process of Redesign

The deliberate and focused process surrounding the subsequent patient care design project spanned about eighteen months. The sequence of events, activities, and accomplishments is described in the following sections.

The Steering Committee

When it became evident that an encompassing initiative to reengineer organizational operations and clinical resource management was required, the executive group created a team to spearhead the task. In an effort to identify innovative and creative people within the organization who demonstrated a commitment to both the organization's stated values and the principles of total quality management, input from staff was sought. An announcement was made in the hospital newsletter, *Vital Signs*, with the request that the names of nominees for the steering committee be forwarded to the president's office. From those identified for possible membership, an interdisciplinary group was structured.

The first tasks of the steering committee included specification of the purpose of the project, its goals, the structure through which the project was to be accomplished, and identification of required resources, including consultation. The primary goals were established: (1) enhancement of patient care, (2) enhancement of quality of work life for staff, and (3) cost reduction of $40 to $50 million (out of a total budget exceeding $240 million). As the meaning of the primary goals was explored, a matrix of principles and elements of change emerged that helped to clarify the parameters of the project.

Three aspects of the organization's mission were specified as important areas for consideration: health care (the delivery of care and services to patients), education, and research. The nature of the organization as an academic medical center necessitated the incorporation of education and research as integral parts of the reengineering since much activity in these areas has a significant impact on care.

Several initiatives were undertaken to ensure that research and education were appropriately involved and considered in the redesign activities. Initially, representation on the steering committee was requested and obtained from the faculties of both medicine and nursing. The intent of this representation was to provide a liaison with both academic groups and to receive input regarding matters of significance to research and education activities and functions. (Later in the project, a group of people concerned about the implications of the project's outcomes for research and education proposed that a subcommittee be formulated to focus on these activities and to promote academic opportunities in each of the design teams. Diverse opinions surrounded the creation of this group. One opinion questioned the advisability of segregating the two functions when the intent of the project was to have *each* design team deliberately focus on research and education in addition to patient care in its assigned area of the organization's operation. Another opinion held that the project represented a unique opportunity to enhance the research and educational capabilities as design proceeded. In the end, the group was constituted as a resource subcommittee with the mandate to provide advice and consultation regarding academic matters within design team activities when warranted and to provide a resource person to each of the design teams.)

The second major task of the steering committee involved the identification of principles to guide the project. In an attempt to communicate to the organization the commitments associated with the project, six major principles were identified: (1) maintenance/ enhancement of the quality of service to patients and of work life for staff, (2) focus on identified patient needs, (3) support for ongoing change and continuing improvement, (4) development of cost-effective alternatives, (5) support for effective relationships, and (6) demonstration of leadership. This beginning thinking on the part of the steering committee paved the way for specific delineation of the operating guidelines and ground rules established to focus project activities.

Purpose

The parameters of the project grew as the steering committee members began to better understand the extent to which redesign was required. In general terms, the purpose was described as follows: "The Patient Care Design Project will manage and facilitate the transition from today's care model to a care model(s) designed to achieve the changes required to respond to the fiscal situation and to ensure quality of care and work life. This will occur through a process which includes widespread consultation and communication with staff" (University of Alberta Hospitals, 1993, p. 2). In this respect, the importance of the alignment among context, infrastructure, and member capability was appreciated as the constraints within the organization related to the delivery of patient care and services were increasingly understood.

Structure

The initial work of the steering committee related to laying the foundation for the project. As exploratory work regarding other organizations' experiences with reengineering was accomplished and as proposals from consulting firms were reviewed, a structure for the project began to take shape in the minds of the members of the steering committee. The structure that emerged is illustrated in Figure 9.2.

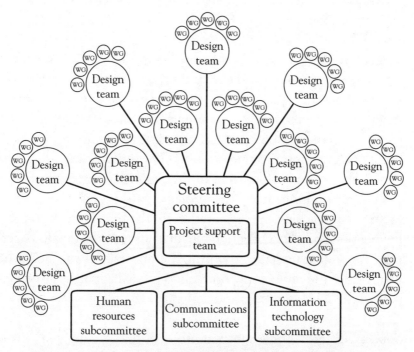

Figure 9.2. Structure of the Patient Care Design Project (WG = "workgroup").

Steering Committee. The steering committee was constituted as the decision-making body for the project. As the broad scope of the project became apparent, members were added to this group to ensure that the appropriate individuals were at the table as the recommendations for change began to emerge. The entire executive team joined the committee and representation from the hospital board was requested; two board members joined the group. Somewhat later, a representative from a partner institution, the Children's Health Center, was added to the group. (The unique collaborative relationship with this organization is described further in Chapter Ten.) Ultimately, membership on the steering committee consisted of administrative and front-line personnel, physicians, other health care professionals, and representatives from the faculties of medicine and nursing at the University of Alberta—a group of about twenty-five people.

Project Support Team. Prior to the beginning of the project, the senior executive group had committed to ensuring adequate operational support for the reengineering process. As a result, about six months into the process, a project support team was appointed. This team consisted of seven members, including an administrative facilitator and an administrative assistant. These individuals were borrowed from their various roles in the organization on a full-time basis for the duration of the project. Initially, the group was involved in readying the organization for the project through communication and data collection plus attending to the details of getting the project under way. During the phases of the project, the members of the project support team provided administrative support to the subcommittees and design teams.

Subcommittees. Three subcommittees of the steering committee were formed several months prior to the commencement of phase I of the project: the human resources subcommittee, the communications subcommittee, and the information technology subcommittee. The role of the human resources subcommittee was to develop innovative and creative strategies for managing staff transition—proactively and in a way that supported the organizational values of respect and partnership. It was recognized from the outset that the changes anticipated would have a pervasive impact on individuals' roles within the organization and that, as a result, some people would no longer have roles. The human resources subcommittee was charged with making this a constructive process to the extent possible. In the initial phase, this subcommittee also attended to the appointment process and educational requirements for the design team leaders and members.

The role of the communications subcommittee was to plan and coordinate the dissemination of information throughout the organization and to stakeholders outside the organization. Members were asked to implement various means of listening to the organizational stakeholders about the ongoing process of the project and to provide regular communication about design activities. In addition, they were asked to develop strategies to assist staff in thinking creatively and generating innovative ideas.

The members of the information technology subcommittee decided early on that the title "information management" would more appropriately describe the role assigned to them. This role included identifying the impact of the design process on information technology, resources, and systems; providing of technical and user advice during the design process; and planning for long-term information technology development based on the care models emerging from the redesign.

Membership on the subcommittees was interdisciplinary with representation from the various departments and levels of the organization. Those selected either volunteered or were nominated to serve on the subcommittees.

Design Teams. The actual reengineering associated with the Patient Care Design Project occurred in design teams and their associated work groups. Design teams were created to focus on specific processes within the organization. Several criteria influenced the naming of design teams. It was important that the processes assigned to each design team be: (1) mutually exclusive yet collectively exhaustive, (2) easily described and explained, (3) manageable, (4) proportional, (5) amenable to interdisciplinary interaction, and (6) open to cross-team integration.

Three types of design teams emerged from a consideration of processes that aligned with the criteria identified above. Eventually, thirteen design teams were chosen encompassing six patient cluster teams, four patient care supply teams, and three patient support teams. These are illustrated in Figure 9.3.

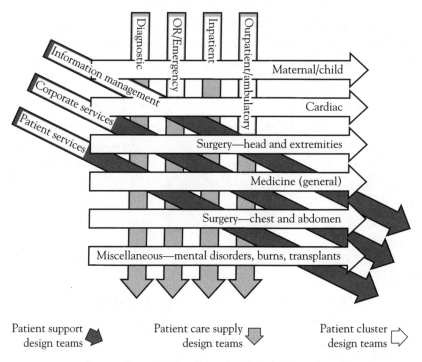

Figure 9.3. Configuration of Design Teams.

Patient cluster design teams were derived from the analysis of data pertaining to the consumption of resources. Patients with similar resource utilization patterns were clustered together. The six clusters generally reflected (1) maternal/child cases, (2) cardiac cases, (3) surgery (head and extremities), (4) medicine (general), (5) surgery (chest and abdomen), and (6) miscellaneous (psychiatry, burns, transplants).

Patient care supply teams were first identified and then tested for manageability and proportionality through the analysis of data. The resulting design teams focused on (1) diagnostic processes, (2) operating room and emergency processes, (3) inpatient processes, and (4) outpatient and ambulatory processes. The patient support design teams were viewed as supplying services to both horizontal (patient cluster) design teams and vertical (patient care supply) design teams. These three dealt with (1) patient services, (2) corporate services, and (3) information management. Each of the thirteen design teams was staffed with fifteen to twenty-five individuals from relevant areas of the hospital's operation. In addition, people with fresh perspectives on the processes being addressed were placed on each design team.

To provide for cross-team liaison and integration as the design phase of the project was under way, representatives from horizontal design teams participated on the vertical design teams. Not only did this serve to unify the work being done by the vertical teams, it provided for communication among the horizontal (patient cluster) design teams.

Consultation

As the steering committee began to appreciate the magnitude of the project being undertaken, it was determined that the assistance of an experienced consultant was required. Although there was significant confidence in the capabilities of individuals within the organization to undertake the task, it was felt that consultation was required to assist with (1) the development and analysis of data, (2) the motivation to adhere to the established time frame, (3) the ability to address problems that had been "not open for discussion" in the past, and (4) as a source of innovative and creative ideas to augment those generated internally.

Although it had not been a practice in the past, the hospital board became involved in the process of selecting a consulting firm to assist with the project. Two major factors contributed to this decision: the political sensitivity of the project and the magnitude of the consulting fees involved. It was determined that a "request for proposal" would be prepared, and a formal search was undertaken.

It was soon determined that only a few consulting firms had personnel who were experienced in the type of reengineering that the hospital was undertaking. The search did not locate any firms that had experience in addressing clinical utilization processes and organizational reengineering simultaneously. One firm was found that had experience far above others with respect to successful restructuring of academic medical centers. The preference was to work with this group: APM Incorporated.

Project Phases

The project consisted of three phases: (1) laying the foundation for redesign, (2) developing restructuring ideas and plans, and (3) implementing the approved ideas and changes. The specific tasks associated with each phase are identified in Figure 9.4.

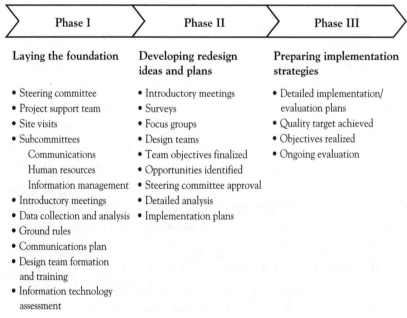

Phase I	Phase II	Phase III
Laying the foundation	**Developing redesign ideas and plans**	**Preparing implementation strategies**
• Steering committee	• Introductory meetings	• Detailed implementation/
• Project support team	• Surveys	evaluation plans
• Site visits	• Focus groups	• Quality target achieved
• Subcommittees	• Design teams	• Objectives realized
Communications	• Team objectives finalized	• Ongoing evaluation
Human resources	• Opportunities identified	
Information management	• Steering committee approval	
• Introductory meetings	• Detailed analysis	
• Data collection and analysis	• Implementation plans	
• Ground rules		
• Communications plan		
• Design team formation and training		
• Information technology assessment		

Figure 9.4. Phases of the Project.

Phase I. Phase I—laying the foundation—included the specification of much of the structure previously described. The project governance was established, principles and guidelines to govern the work were articulated, and design teams were named based on an analysis of data and processes. People were selected to lead and to participate in design teams, training was provided, and, based on preliminary data and the experience of the consultant elsewhere, the design teams were assigned targets related to the improvement of care processes, work life enhancement, and cost reduction.

Phase II. Phase II consisted of the development of redesign ideas and plans. It began with design team activity and concluded with the development of implementation plans for the approved ideas for reengineering. As design teams became familiar with their particular areas of focus, they were supported administratively by a member of the project support team, a data analyst, and a consultant. Each team also had an executive champion whose role was to encourage the grappling with "thorny issues" and assist in the removal of barriers as they were encountered.

The work of the design teams was enhanced by work groups that were spawned as specific initiatives and opportunities were identified and detailed analysis and work on them were required. As recommendations for change were identified and developed, they were taken to the steering committee for approval. From there coordinated plans for implementation of clinical utilization improvements and organizational reengineering initiatives were developed.

Phase III. Phase III pertained to the implementation of change initiatives with the creation of a system to coordinate initiatives and monitor the changes. Less complex changes were implemented first, with more detailed planning occurring for the more complex ideas.

It was anticipated that the project would lead to an ongoing process of review and redesign, with continuous improvement of existing processes occurring simultaneously with significant reengineering initiatives.

Project Outcomes

The commitment of the organization to redesign both clinical resource utilization and organizational operations provided new and meaningful opportunities for unique customized innovation. The design teams were created in a manner that focused the outcomes directly on the requirements of the patients. The patient cluster teams defined "best practice" by assessing the appropriateness of interventions for addressing "needs" as outlined in care maps. Patient care supply teams then responded by providing the required supplies and services. In turn, once the needs of the patient cluster and patient care design teams were established, the three patient support teams developed structures and processes to support the defined activity. Thus, the outcomes of the entire process were focused primarily on the needs of the patients through meaningful customer-supplier relationships.

As this chapter was being written, the Patient Care Design Project was in Phase II—the interdisciplinary design teams were working on generating issues; evaluating their impact on quality of care, work life, and resources; and planning for the implementation of change initiatives. The specific outcomes were yet to emerge. There were, however, areas of anticipated change based on the early work of the design teams and the understanding of the experiences and outcomes of other organizations' redesign initiatives.

One of the most significant early outcomes related to the organizational context: at the outset of Phase II, the need to revisit the strategic operating vision became apparent.

In the months preceding the project, some uncertainty had developed within the organization regarding the strategic vision of the hospital. This was related to regional discussions surrounding relocation of services and consolidation of hospitals. For a time, hospital officials took a nonprotectionist, systemic position with respect to regionalization and rationalization. This stance, although perceived to be in the best interest of the system, created uncertainty on the part of the board, the academics/physicians, and the staff about the integrity and viability of the hospital as an academic health center. In addition, as the magnitude and potential impact of the Patient Care Design Project came to be appreciated within the organization, so did the necessity for a renewed strategic vision to obtain staff commitment and provide direction for the clinical and organizational redesign.

These two factors prompted the hospital's board to initiate a process to develop a renewed vision and strategic direction for the hospital. The board, working with the department chairs, declared: "The University Hospital is a leading academic, research, and patient care center offering a wide range of services and programs. The University Hospital Board is committed to work with others, with respect and in partnership, to provide a health system for the benefit of Albertans, today and in the future" (University of Alberta Hospitals, 1994). This became an important "stake in the ground," both for the project and for the evolution of the regional design of the health care system.

Since Phase II was incomplete when this chapter was written, anticipated infrastructure changes presented in the following section are based on early discussions within the design teams and knowledge of other organizations' experiences.

There was commitment within the hospital to initiate changes in patient aggregation and work distribution based on commonality of resource requirements. The development of care maps and the use of clinical practice guidelines were developed to enhance quality and efficiency with respect to designing care processes and defining the specific service requirements of patient groups.

The redesign of clinical processes and the definition of service, supply, and support requirements would lead to staffing innovations, such as the creation of new roles, the cross-training of members of professional disciplines and of support workers, and the refinement of the management and administrative support requirements for the ongoing work of the organization. In addition, the project presented the opportunity to address long-standing architectural issues related to unit size and staffing levels.

The redesigning of clinical resource management and the reengineering of institutional operations posed significant challenges for the academic organizations associated with the hospital. For this reason, representatives from the relevant university faculties participated in the design team process. Teaching and research programs must be aligned and compatible with the quality of care, quality of work life, and cost reduction initiatives undertaken as part of the redesign. For many, this alignment will result in a significant and difficult paradigm shift of an unprecedented nature.

Sizable resources will be required in "enabling initiatives," particularly as related to information technology. As specific ideas for change emerge, there will be the opportunity to invest some of the savings in technology that will promote further efficiency and effectiveness.

Lessons Learned

Although the Patient Care Design Project was still in progress at the time this chapter was written, lessons had emerged throughout the foundational year leading up to the intense activity associated with the redesign process in Phase II. As with other major projects reported in this book, the lessons learned can be viewed in terms of the three domains of the Organization Capability Development Framework.

Context

The context, as the domain within which the parameters for the project were set, required careful attention. Obviously, the context for the entire project was the organizational context as it related to total quality management. However, the project itself required a context that would create the specific environment and direction for the changes that were to be created. Specification of the purpose of the redesign initiative, the vision of the organization, and the operating guidelines and ground rules for design activities all contributed to the success of the project.

Purpose. It was important from the outset to delineate the purpose of the initiative. The stated organizational goals related to quality of patient care, quality of work life, and financial targets were repeatedly referred to as the redesign activities proceeded.

Strategic Operating Vision. It became clear, as organizational members became familiar with the intent and process associated with the project, that a better understanding of the preferred future for the hospital was required to provide both direction and destination for the design teams and work groups. Accordingly, a task group consisting of board members, department chairs, and the executive team was commissioned to update the strategic operating vision of the hospital. The outcome of this activity was a crystallized and concise picture envisioned for the organization as the regionalization and rationalization of the health care system emerged. It was felt that by clearly describing this strategic vision, the ability to create the future rather than merely respond to it would be enhanced. As well, the vision became a guide for both the redesign activities and budgetary adjustments that became necessary in the course of events.

Operating Guidelines. Operating guidelines were established to provide direction to team members as to what questions needed to be addressed in determining the redesign initiatives. Five questions served to cluster the considerations: (1) What work (how much) should be done? (2) When should the work be done? (3) How should the work be done? (4) Who should do the work? and

(5) Where should the work be done? The following list illustrates additional topics related to each of the questions.

What (how much) work should be done?
- define best practice
- consider continuum of care
- base level of care on clinical needs
- reduce/eliminate nonessential activities
- change products/services

When should the work be done?
- consider timeliness and urgency
- consider best time for patient
- consider patient need
- do work when it is least costly

How should the work be done?
- minimize variation
- streamline processes
- use enabling technology

Who should do the work?
- involve patients/customers/suppliers
- determine "in-house" versus "contract" appropriateness
- redefine roles/interrelationships
  - team approach • centralize/decentralize • broaden job responsibilities • align accountability/authority/responsibility • staff to demand • delegate work to most cost-effective, appropriately trained worker

Where should the work be done?
- move resources to patients
- optimize physical facilities
- align services with mission/vision

The operating guidelines were constructed to empower the members of the design teams to challenge formerly unquestioned practices associated with the delivery of care. Design teams were instructed to "use these guidelines to conduct a fundamental and objective review of processes to achieve sustainable breakthrough improvements in the way patient care, education, and research are delivered, at the same or better level of quality and service with significantly reduced cost and time."

Ground Rules. Where the operating principles addressed the "what" of the design team and work group processes, the ground rules addressed the "how" by defining the parameters that guided the functioning within the groups. All members of the design teams were expected to adhere to the ground rules; through this process, the discussions and considerations were facilitated, enhanced, and strengthened, and it was possible to address issues that in the past had not been open for discussion.

Infrastructure

With respect to the infrastructure associated with the project, two major areas of consideration were vital to the success of the project: communication within the organization, and the processes and structures related to the design teams.

Communication. Even prior to the initiation of the project, it was apparent from examining other organizations' experiences in redesign and from discussions with consultants that there could never be enough communication with the organizational members. The steering committee members were committed to providing extensive, comprehensive communication repeated through a multitude of forms of media to ensure that information about the process and outcomes of the project was readily available.

Another challenge was the communication required among the various groups associated with the project: steering committee, subcommittees, project support team, consultants, design teams, and work groups. To facilitate this, a leadership forum was structured to provide for liaison among the design teams and the steering committee. Through this mechanism, design team leaders were able to stay abreast of the activities of the other teams. In addition, liaison members from each of the patient cluster design teams participated as members of the vertical and diagonal design teams to provide for "cross-pollination" at yet another level of activity.

Scheduling. Even before the design team activity began, there was recognition that the scheduling of meetings would be a challenge. Several initiatives were undertaken to assist. A request went out to organizational members from the chief executive that, where possible, regular organizational activities be suspended for the duration of the design team phase. Second, a schedule of design team meetings was formulated to ensure consistent timing of meetings. This was particularly important for support team members and for those who were functioning in liaison activities.

As much as a consistent schedule was important to maintain coordination of activities and support for the teams' work, it was also necessary to be flexible and adaptable in the event that all did not go as planned. This was especially important when major events in the phasing schedule did not proceed as anticipated. Resilience in the face of complications prevented frustration and helped focus energy on the constructive activity of the project. As it turned out, the phases did not proceed exactly as scheduled. However, more often than not, delays actually enhanced the ability to proceed effectively with the subsequent steps of the redesign effort.

Design Team Structure. The structure of the design teams was another important element associated with the infrastructure. The commitment was made early in the project to provide a significant amount of support for design team activity. Each of the teams was supported by a member of the project support team, a consultant, an analyst from the hospital, and an executive champion. Team leaders and coleaders were appointed on the basis of their demonstrated interest in and commitment to total quality management and the organization. It was possible to appoint a physician coleader to each team, and in most situations, this person was the clinical expert in the area of focus for the design team. The process leader for the group tended to be more remote from the particular area under consideration; it was hoped that this would enhance objectivity and creativity. The executive champions were appointed on the basis of their noninvolvement in the area. When untouchable issues were encountered, the executives were expected to negotiate with their colleagues in the executive team to ensure that any barriers were removed.

It was recognized that, for some members of the organization to participate, relief staff would be required. As a result, policies were developed to permit access to relief funding if job responsibilities required ongoing and consistent activity. Money was set aside in the project budget so that this support would not be taken directly from the cost centers in functional units.

Member Capability

Member capability pertains to the knowledge, skills, and commitment of those within the organization. Of particular importance in this project were the involvement of physicians and the training provided for design team members.

Physician Involvement. It was evident at the outset of the project that its success depended largely on the extent to which physicians became involved, particularly since the focus of the initiative rested on the work of the patient cluster design teams relative to the development of "best practice" guidelines. Several steps were taken to achieve the commitment of physicians, some of which were based on Wensel's (1993, p. 90) "tips" for involving physicians and clinical staff in quality improvement activities. In particular, meetings were planned at times convenient to medical staff (late afternoon), time commitments were minimal and clear, and meeting agendas were well planned and succinct. Emphasis was placed on improving care and on the partnerships of hospital staff and physicians. Additionally, attention was directed to flawed processes rather than to individuals' practice.

Training. A firm foundation of capability was required by design team members. Comprehensive information about the reason for the project, its purpose, parameters, and process formed the content of educational sessions. Team leaders were provided with information about the context of the project, capability in effectively leading groups and analytical processes, and expectations surrounding functioning in the role. Team members received a somewhat abbreviated version. In the foundational phase of the project, the members of the project support team were equipped with the capability required for the facilitative role they would play.

Consultation. As was mentioned before, it was determined early in the project that assistance from an outside source was required to enable the organization to proceed expeditiously with the project. Although there was significant confidence in the capabilities of organizational members, it was recognized that this was the first major reengineering effort that had ever been undertaken within the hospital. The lack of experience within the organization necessitated consultation with an outside source. The involvement of the consultants from APM Incorporated was of great value; they contributed significantly to the progress and outcome of the initiative.

A Project in Progress

Hammer and Champy (1993, p. 46) define reengineering as "the fundamental rethinking and radical redesign of business processes to achieve dramatic improvements in critical, contemporary, measures of performance." Such was the commitment for the Patient Care Design Project.

At the point of publication of this book, the project was incomplete. Although many significant changes were emerging, the total impact of the reengineering of clinical utilization and the subsequent organizational redesign had not yet evolved. However, much was learned in the beginning phases of the redesign. This chapter has provided the reader with an overview of the issues that contributed to the initiation of the project, a detailed description of the process and structure associated with the redesign, beginning understandings related to project outcomes, and the lessons that emerged even as the foundational and beginning design work was undertaken.

References

Andrews, H. A., and Wensel, R. H. "Promoting Physician-Nurse Collaboration Throughout the Organization." *Healthcare Management FORUM*, 1992, 5(4), 28–33.

Berwick, D. M., and Plsek, P. E. "Managing Medical Quality." In J. Brill (ed.), *Program One: The Need and the Opportunity*. Woodbridge, N.J.: Visions, 1992.

Curran, C. "Changing the Way We Do Business." *Nursing Economic$*, 1991, 9(5), 296.

Hammer, M., and Champy, J. *Reengineering the Corporation: A Manifesto for Business Revolution*. New York: HarperCollins, 1993.

Lathrop, J. P. "Where Your Wage Dollar Goes." *Healthcare Forum Journal*, July/August 1991, p. 18.

University of Alberta Hospitals. Presentation materials, Patient Care Design Project. Edmonton: University of Alberta Hospitals, 1993.

University of Alberta Hospitals. *Newsflash*. Edmonton: University of Alberta Hospitals, 1994.

Wensel, R. H. "Tips for Involving Professional Staff in CQI." In M. Harrigan (ed.), *Quest for Quality in Canadian Health Care*. Ottawa: Minister of Supply and Services Canada, 1993.

Chapter Ten

Collaboration: Working with Partners

Janet M. Davidson

The previous chapters have described the major initiatives undertaken by the University of Alberta Hospital as part of the organizational transformation process and the context in which those initiatives took place. On reading these chapters, it becomes evident that responsibility for the success of these initiatives (or lack of it) did not rest solely with the hospital but rather was a shared responsibility among a variety of collaborators or partners. The success of any particular strategy was due in large measure to the degree to which the hospital was able to forge positive and meaningful partnerships with interested and committed stakeholders.

Just as partnership is an important value within an individual organization, effective collaboration—both internal and external—is also important to the success of the system overall. For example, by working together acute care hospitals and long-term–care facilities can ensure an integrated and coordinated discharge planning process that facilitates the appropriate placement of long-term–care patients, thus resulting in a more effective and efficient use of increasingly limited health care dollars—in short, a better-quality system. As the hospital's chief executive described in an interview for the Canadian Health Development Foundation,

> In August 1992 the Conference of Deputy Ministers called together
> a number of people to voice a different vision for the operation of
> the health care system. The statement that emerged emphasized

consumer-centered quality that makes Canada a global leader in health care. It is the collaboration of all the constituents that underlines its quality (Langlois and Schurman, 1993, p. 3).

The Value of Partnership

Chapter Three included a discussion of the University of Alberta Hospital's vision statement and the critical importance of effective partnerships in that vision. Partnership is also one of the hospital's three core values, along with respect and continuous improvement. In developing these core values, it was realized that the ability to achieve the vision was dependent, in large measure, on an ability to forge meaningful partnerships with appropriate groups—patients, employees, educational institutions, government, suppliers, and other health care providers, to name only a few. For the hospital staff members, a commitment to the core value of partnership meant more than simply collaboration or sharing. It meant being committed to one another's success—"your success is my success."

Collaboration through effective partnerships is critical to the success of any organization. In this period of major restructuring in health care systems worldwide, effective partnerships are becoming a distinguishing characteristic of success. As Krackhardt (1992, p. 238) notes,

> If change were simply dependent on new information, then weak ties would be preeminent. But when it comes to major change, change that may threaten the status quo in terms of power and the standard routines of how decisions are made, then resistance to that change must be addressed before predictions can be made about the success of that change effort. A major resource that is required to bring about such change is trust in the propagators of that change. Change is the product of strong, effective, and time-honoured relationships.

What do effective partnerships look like? Or, alternatively, how can one tell when a partnership is not working? First and foremost, it is important to recognize that an effective partnership is much more than just an agreement (written or otherwise). Successful partnerships are as much a result of the "how" as the "what" associated with the collaboration. For example, collective agreements define the nature (the "what") of relationships between unionized employees and management. However, anyone who has been involved in labor-management issues knows full well that even the best of collective agreements can only go so far in promoting a collaborative partnership. What is needed is a strong commitment among all participants to a shared vision and to one another.

Another example is the relationship between individual hospitals and government. The "what" of this relationship is explained at length in various pieces of legislation and accompanying regulations as well as in a multitude of policies and directives. However, despite these attempts, most would agree that the process associated with the relationship—the "how"—between the two parties is fair at best. Both "sides" are highly suspicious of each other, with little commitment to a common vision or to each other's success.

By focusing on the "how" of relationships, members of the hospital's executive group are learning many lessons about effective collaboration to enhance relationships with their partners. Some examples are success stories; others point to the need for improvement and continued work.

Examples of Collaboration with Partners

The University of Alberta Hospital has been involved in a number of partnership initiatives in recent years as part of its organizational transformation initiative. These partnership efforts have involved the local community, government, other health care organizations, employees, and other stakeholders.

Local Community

In the early 1990s, the University of Alberta Hospital was designated one of the province's four major trauma centers. To support this role and to facilitate quick and easy access to the hospital's sophisticated resources, it was concluded that construction of a licensed heliport facility was required.

Existing arrangements required that patients be transferred to the hospital either by ground ambulance or, in an extreme emergency, by helicopter to an adjacent field on the University of Alberta campus, and then by surface transport the one-block distance to the hospital emergency department. This practice was not considered appropriate from a patient care point of view. It was also a source of frustration for some local residents. Concerned about the level of noise and its potentially adverse effects on the quality of life in the community, they expressed opposition to any role for the hospital that would necessitate aircraft landing in the area.

As soon as the hospital board gave its approval to plan for and construct a heliport, an open letter was sent to the community leagues in the four surrounding neighborhoods advising them of the hospital's intentions and seeking their input into the development of a heliport site that would best meet the interests and concerns of both groups. Open meetings were also scheduled with the four groups to explain the hospital's need for a heliport and to listen to residents' concerns. Tours were arranged for residents to visit some of the hospital's critical care areas, such as the neonatal, burn, and trauma intensive care units, to give them a better understanding of the hospital's role as a trauma center. Local area residents were also invited to participate in noise studies and to provide input into the review of the various siting alternatives.

The majority of residents expressed satisfaction with the proactive approach the hospital board and administrative staff had taken in trying to arrive at a solution that was acceptable to all concerned. However, a small, vocal group of residents remained opposed and took official steps to block approval of the project by the city of Edmonton. In an effort to resolve the situation, a "last ditch" effort was made to meet with these individuals on the evening before the city was to make its decision. Members of the hospital board, senior administration, medical staff, and air ambulance personnel attended an open meeting and once again explained the hospital's position. Detailed information on anticipated helicopter activity and proposed flight paths was provided. As well, the hospital administration made a commitment to keep the community informed of any significant changes to the projected helicopter activity or flight paths. A commitment was also made to establish a community liaison committee composed of representatives from each of the four community leagues and the hospital that would meet regularly to discuss issues of mutual interest and concern.

The outcome of these efforts was an official withdrawal of the residents' objection to the project. A rooftop heliport was constructed and officially opened ten months later. The community liaison committee has been meeting regularly with community representatives for over a year, and members have expressed satisfaction at the opportunity to share information with a major partner in their community.

Government

In late 1992, representatives of Alberta's Department of Health (Public Health Division) formally approached the University of Alberta Hospital regarding the transfer of responsibility for the Provincial Laboratory of Public Health for Northern Alberta (PLPHNA) from the University of Alberta to the hospital. This formal approach was preceded by a series of informal discussions, initiated by the hospital, that attempted to clarify for government the hospital's interest in expanding its role in public health.

Given that the hospital's own laboratory had recently assumed a major role in public health water testing and that the PLPHNA was housed in the same building as the hospital's laboratory facilities, with close service and staff linkages between the two, it was deemed appropriate to investigate the possibility of placing both laboratory facilities under the same management structure. It was believed that such a reorganization would result in improved service quality at reduced cost.

A committee was established under the chairmanship of the Division of Public Health that included representatives from the University of Alberta, the University of Alberta Hospital, the Government of Alberta, and the PLPHNA. This group was charged with identifying the various management options for the PLPHNA, examining the advantages and disadvantages of each from the perspective of each stakeholder, and recommending a course of action to government.

This committee met regularly over the course of almost a year and developed a comprehensive transfer plan that attempted to address the interests and concerns of all parties. Of particular concern were issues related to the transfer of staff from the university to the hospital. Considerable time and effort, therefore, was devoted to meeting with union representatives and to arriving at solutions that were acceptable to the majority of the staff involved. The committee's report was submitted and approved; the transfer took place shortly thereafter.

The success of this partnership initiative can perhaps best be summed up in the words of the Minister of Health in her letter to the hospital's chief executive following the transfer:

> I am pleased to hear of the successful transfer for the administration
> of the Provincial Laboratory for Public Health for Northern Alberta.
> . . . I understand that this important change occurred smoothly,
> thanks to the commitment and competent effort of a number of significant players. I would like to express my appreciation to you, Don,
> for your support in this process and acknowledge the contribution
> of several members of your staff who were instrumental in the suc-

cess of the transfer. . . . Each of these persons made a special contribution to the success of this initiative and I would ask that you express my personal thanks to them for a job well done (S. McClellan, letter to the chief executive, August 24, 1993).

Other Health Care Organizations

In the late 1980s, the University of Alberta Hospital initiated a strategic planning process aimed at clarifying its role as an academic medical center. A by-product of this process was a thorough review of the hospital's general long-term–care programs and services, which resulted in a decision by the hospital board to divest itself of these responsibilities. The board concluded that, given the hospital's focus on acute care, long-term–care patients and the staff involved in caring for them would be better served by an organization whose primary focus was long-term care.

Given the hospital's long-standing role in long-term care and recognizing that the transfer of such programs was a complex and potentially sensitive matter, it was determined that, rather than attempting to negotiate a transfer of all the long-term–care programs at once, it would be best to proceed on a component-by-component basis, commencing with the Mewburn Veterans Centre (MVC). The MVC is a 146-bed, long-term–care facility dedicated to the provision of continuing care to residents—primarily male—who meet eligibility criteria established by Veterans Affairs Canada. Initially established by the federal government, with funding provided by the provincial government, and actively supported by local war veterans' groups, the MVC represented a unique challenge in the arena of program transfers. Complicating the matter further was the fact that the land on which the MVC stood was owned by another hospital board.

Nonetheless, the hospital's senior administrators began looking for potential partners for this transfer. In the summer of 1992, they approached the Capital Care Group, a publicly owned organization committed to excellence in continuing care, with the proposal that it assume responsibility for operating the MVC. It was felt that a transfer to the Capital Care Group had the best potential for success, given the strong mutual commitment of both organizations to service quality. The Capital Care Group agreed to this request, and a transfer planning committee was established with representatives from both the hospital and the Capital Care Group, as well as from the Alberta Department of Health. Both organizations recognized the importance of success with this transfer venture as it could serve as a model for future similar transfers within the province.

At the outset, both organizations agreed that the fundamental reason for the transfer must be the best interest of the patients. To that end, they established six principles that would serve as the basis for all transfer planning: (1) that the long-term–care expertise of the Capital Care Group be maximized to benefit residents and their families, (2) that adverse impacts on existing staff be minimized, (3) that there be no decrease in the long-term–care bed complement in the Edmonton region, (4) that the Capital Care Group operate the MVC within the available funding, (5) that there be a cooperative and conjoint communication strategy and plan for all internal and external stakeholders, and (6) that all regulatory and other requirements of the Government of Alberta and Veterans Affairs Canada be met.

In addition to the transfer planning committee, which met monthly, each organization established its own project transfer team that was responsible for managing the day-to-day details related to the transfer. A bridging committee also was established to keep residents and their families, as well as staff, fully informed about what was taking place and to assist in allaying their fears. This committee provided an opportunity for staff and residents to have input into key decisions affecting their futures. These meetings were complemented with a variety of informal information exchanges and regular newsletters. The emphasis was on open and honest communication among all concerned.

The two issues that were pivotal to the potential success (or failure) of the transfer were: (1) the differing organizational cultures and (2) the different collective agreements with the unions. With respect to organizational culture, hospital staff were concerned that many of the benefits of the hospital's total quality management environment would be lost to them if and when they moved to the Capital Care Group. When these concerns were brought to the attention of the Capital Care Group administrators, they met with the staff to discuss ways in which these concerns could be addressed. One strategy that was implemented as a result of these discussions was that the Capital Care Group agreed to maintain the self-directed work teams in place at the MVC even though this was not a practice in any of its other facilities.

Dealing with the differing collective agreements with the unions required tireless effort on the part of human resources staff in both organizations to ensure that staff were not disadvantaged as a result of the transfer. Both organizations had a history of positive and productive relationships with their respective unions, which aided the transfer process considerably. The entire transfer process took approximately ten months and was seen by all concerned to be a model for future transfers.

A few months later, another transfer of the general long-term–care program between the hospital and the Capital Care Group was undertaken. Regrettably, this transfer did not proceed as smoothly. Many of the issues that arose during this second transfer were not entirely within the control of the two organizations. For example, because a number of their members had been laid off as a result of funding cuts, the unions in the Capital Care Group would not agree to recognize the seniority rights of hospital staff who would potentially be transferred with the program. As a result, most staff chose not to transfer and the hospital was forced to institute layoff procedures. At the completion of the first transfer, if the two organizations had carried out a thorough analysis of all the factors contributing to its success, the problems that arose with the second transfer might have been anticipated and appropriate corrective action taken.

Employees

At the time the University of Alberta Hospital commenced the quality journey, efforts were focused on improving care for the primary customer, the patient. Many efforts looked at ways in which patient satisfaction could be increased. Over the years, the members of the senior executive team came to appreciate the fact that high-quality patient care is, among other things, a product of satisfied and motivated employees.

With that recognition, it became apparent that ways to increase employee satisfaction needed to be examined. A commitment was made to involve staff more actively in "running" the institution—to treating them as important partners. In earlier chapters, a number of partnership arrangements with staff were described, in particular the C.A.R.E. Governance Model and the development of a new management performance and compensation system. There was a wide variety of other initiatives, only a few of which are described here.

The members of the hospital board and administration have long realized that the hospital's ability to carry out its role in a cost-effective and efficient manner and to deliver high-quality patient care is highly dependent on the staff. This awareness required an examination of the relationships with employee groups and their unions with a view to forging more positive partnerships.

As noted earlier, the hospital was well known for having open and cooperative relationships with its employee unions. This was evidenced by the fact that the hospital—at the request of its unions—was one of the few in the province that bargained directly with unions rather than through the bargaining process managed by the Alberta Healthcare Association on behalf of the majority of hospitals. That is not to say that issues and concerns did not arise. However, there was a general recognition that the problems that did exist were not the result of any lack of commitment on any one group's part.

The University of Alberta Hospital undertook a number of initiatives to meaningfully involve the unions in the decision-making structure of the hospital. At one point, it was felt that forging relationships with staff members, individually and collectively, would appropriately link with the unions, but this proved to be an erroneous assumption. The individual employees were not in a position to relay the opinions of their unions nor were the unions prepared to have individuals who were not in official roles speak on their behalf.

As was described in Chapter Five and mentioned earlier in this chapter, official union involvement was requested in both the first implementation of a nursing governance structure and the development of the second. Although the union representatives contributed significantly to both of these initiatives and their support was highly valued, problems occurred when all did not run smoothly. In both instances of implementation—the first attempt and the C.A.R.E. Governance Model—the decision of the union to withdraw its support and to advise its members to not participate confused the organization and eventually led the hospital to abandon the model in favor of the professional advisory committee structure involving all disciplines.

Union involvement in the hospital's President's Council was another case in point. In an attempt to forge meaningful relationships with the hospital's unions, the elected heads of the union locals were invited to sit as voting members of the President's Council—the hospital's senior administrative decision-making forum. It soon became apparent that this arrangement was not satisfactory from either a union or a hospital perspective.

Union officials believed that decisions were already *faits accomplis* before the issues were presented for discussion at the council. Hospital administrators were frustrated at the union officials' lack of input into the decisions. In mutual analysis of the problem, it became apparent that the decision-making processes of the organizations were in conflict. Where the hospital officials at the table were the senior administrators in the hospital and were empowered to make decisions on behalf of the organization, the union representatives, as elected officials, were expected to consult their membership on matters of concern and were not empowered to take a position on behalf of their unions. With this discrepancy, the effectiveness of the President's Council was compromised. The invitation for union participation was withdrawn and the former structure was resumed.

Nonetheless, the commitment to effective involvement of unions in the hospital continued. There were ongoing attempts to enhance the partnerships with these important stakeholders. In recent years, a number of retreats bringing together hospital managers and union representatives have been held to clarify respective roles, responsibilities, and expectations and to identify strategies for improving relationships. Furthermore, union-specific labor-management forums have been established to address any and all issues related to terms and conditions of employment for each of the employee groups. As well, there are regular (quarterly) meetings between the hospital's senior executives and union officials to discuss issues and to keep each other informed on major initiatives.

Prior to the last two rounds of negotiations, the hospital and union negotiating teams participated in team-building retreats to enhance and facilitate the bargaining process. In the 1994 negotiations, all parties expressed a commitment to undertake "mutual gains" bargaining. In this framework, the teams mutually develop solutions to issues rather than forging agreements from significantly polarized positions.

The hospital and its unions continue to be committed to effective partnerships. It was helpful for hospital officials to come to an understanding that the mandates and commitments of the organizations do not always coincide. Where the hospital's mandate is primarily the provision of quality patient care, the unions exist primarily to forge and protect "rights" for their members, although a commitment to quality patient care from the unions' perspectives would also be espoused. The understanding of this reality has assisted hospital officials in determining appropriate, effective, and meaningful avenues for involvement.

The University

As described in Chapter One, the University of Alberta Hospital is situated on the campus of the University of Alberta, Canada's second-largest university. Although the two institutions are completely autonomous, with separate boards, administrations, and separate pieces of legislation governing their operations, there is a long-standing tradition of close collaboration. Indeed, the dean of the faculty of medicine and the university's president are members of the hospital board.

With the construction of the Walter C. Mackenzie Health Sciences Centre—the hospital's newest facility—the need for close linkages with the health sciences faculties was explicitly recognized by incorporating the faculty of medicine administration and many faculty offices, as well as the University of Alberta's health sciences library, within the center. Additionally, the faculty of nursing is in a building adjacent to and connected with the center, as are the medical research facilities. Cross-appointments, particularly between these two faculties and the hospital, are the order of the day. In the case of the faculty of medicine, all faculty chairs of clinical departments (with two exceptions) are also the hospital's departmental chairs. As a routine, the hospital administration is involved in the search-and-selection process for most of the key positions on the faculty.

In recognition of the need to establish more formal linkages between the two organizations, in the mid-1980s an affiliation agreement was developed that, among other things, outlined the nature of the relationship, provided for cross-leasing and other facility-sharing arrangements (basically each organization agreed to share facilities with the other at no cost), and established a process for close collaboration among all of the health sciences faculties at the university and their corresponding departments at the hospital. Currently, the two organizations are working together to establish a research affiliation agreement. This is proving to be a challenging process in view of the rights and interests of both organizations with respect to intellectual property. However, both organizations have agreed that the primary objective of any agreement of this type is to facilitate high-quality research. Given the alignment around that objective, there is confidence that the concerns of both organizations can be addressed satisfactorily.

A wide variety of mechanisms has been put into place to facilitate the ongoing, day-to-day collaboration between the two organizations. For example, a Medical Center Coordinating Committee, composed of the dean of medicine, the associate deans, and the hospital's president and vice presidents, meets monthly to discuss issues of common concern. The committee addresses matters such as faculty appointments, residency training, and physician manpower planning. Another example is the hospital's Special Services and Research Committee—a committee of the hospital board responsible for approving all research conducted in the hospital—which is chaired by the dean of medicine and includes representation from both the hospital and the university. There are also close linkages to the university's ethics review processes. The hospital has entered into a number of collaborative ventures with the faculty of medicine including (with another partner, the Alberta Asthma Foundation) the establishment of the Alberta Asthma Center, which has as its mandate the support of education, research, and treatment initiatives in asthma care. There are also efforts underway to establish a joint health care outcomes research center.

Other Partnerships

There are myriad other examples of collaborative partnerships that the hospital has established with its stakeholders. These include, for example, equipment servicing agreements, care provision agreements, and product development initiatives.

Equipment Servicing. The University of Alberta Hospital has one of the largest clinical engineering departments of any hospital in the country. Other hospitals have entered into agreements with the University of Alberta Hospital's clinical engineering department to service some of their equipment rather than have it serviced by suppliers that may not have any locally based service staff. This arrangement allows the other hospitals access to immediate service by people who know their institution and equipment.

From the University of Alberta Hospital's point of view, the service agreements provide a source of revenue that allows it to maintain a full complement of highly trained clinical engineers. The hospital also has entered into a variety of similar service agreements with local area hospitals for the provision of food and laundry services.

Care Provision: Pediatric Services. The hospital has entered into an agreement with the Children's Health Center, an organization with a distinct board and administrative structure charged with delivering health care to children in the northern half of the province. The agreement calls for the consolidation of inpatient pediatric services at the Walter C. Mackenzie Health Sciences Centre. This partnership has the advantage of improving quality of care for children by consolidating most services at one site. At the same time, it improves cost-efficiency in the system by utilizing existing resources rather than requiring the construction of a separate facility for children.

Product Development. The hospital has, particularly in recent years, become involved in a number of partnerships with product developers. These partnerships have ranged from working with particular manufacturers in the development and testing of new medical devices, such as infusion pumps and respirators, to working with researchers/scientists in the development of new food products. All of these efforts have proven to be learning experiences for both the hospital and its collaborators.

Lessons Learned

On analysis of the keys to success in effective collaborative relationships with partners, specific themes emerged. They related to the three domains of the Organization Capability Development Framework: context, infrastructure, and member capability.

Context

The context of the organization was described in Chapter Two as the components that create the environment in which organizational activities take place—the mission, vision, values, and principles. Successful outcomes in the hospital's collaboration with partners related particularly to the mutual understanding of mission and objectives that emerged as a result of involvement and interaction. In addition, the principles and ground rules associated with effective relationships set important parameters for the relationships.

It was important to understand and respect that different organizations have different mandates and missions. These differences may inhibit the extent to which any one partner can engage in the collaboration. The hospital's aim may be efficient, cost-effective management of hospital resources, while a supplier partner has an important profit motive. Unions' mandates relate to the job security and benefits of their members; the hospital's actions may compromise the union's ability to achieve that, particularly in a time of fiscal constraint.

Another understanding pertained to one of the management principles developed by the hospital's executive: collaboration. To quote the hospital's Management Statement (University of Alberta Hospitals, 1993),

> Collaborating means listening to and, if appropriate, acting upon the concerns and contributions of others in accomplishing the work. It does not mean consensus or universal agreement. Rather, collaboration means involvement and inclusion of others in the design and coordination of work.

Prior to achieving this understanding, there was confusion within the hospital as attempts were made to empower staff and decentralize decision making. The importance of clarifying the party responsible for making the actual decision has helped refine the process of collaboration. For this reason, it was imperative that principles of relationships and terms of reference for specific forums be mutually developed and understood. Such clarity in the partnership promoted the ability to work together effectively and in a mutually beneficial way.

The ground rules associated with effective relationships as described in Chapter Four continued to be the key to effective collaboration with the hospital's partners. Committed speaking and listening and the associated ground rules of effective relationships were demonstrated repeatedly to be key in the development of productive and effective relational processes.

Although all partners did not feel comfortable committing to the ground rules of effective relationships, these were prominent in every interaction—posted on meeting room walls, printed on meeting agendas—and hospital personnel were conscientious in their attempts to continually adhere to their intent. This provided the partners in the relationship a visible and clear understanding of the hospital's intent in the relationship.

Infrastructure

Infrastructure was described earlier as the systems, processes, and procedures—relational, technical, and developmental—within which work gets done. The infrastructure associated with the hospital's partnership arrangements pertained to the specific linkages that were created to promote consistent communication, issue resolution, and joint initiatives.

The hospital found it vital to have specific forums and structures in place to provide for this linkage. For example, several regularly scheduled meetings of various representatives of the unions' executive with hospital personnel were successful in addressing particular matters of mutual concern. In the partnership with the Children's Health Center, a pediatric management committee was created to attend to the issues arising throughout the consolidation. In addition, reciprocal appointment of two board members to the other institution's board of directors served to provide the required linkage at the governance level.

In many partnership arrangements, personnel dedicated to the nurturance of the relationship proved to be beneficial. In the union-management forums, one vice president was appointed to be the link with the unions' executive. One contributor to the success of the transfer of the long-term–care program at the MVC was the appointment of a designated person responsible for the coordination of the negotiations. The hospital continues to strive to ensure that designated individuals assume ownership for collaborative initiatives; when problems have occurred, they have often been the result of this structural factor having been neglected.

It became evident that specific linkages throughout the organization were required for successful collaboration with partners. A consistent challenge in relationships with unions was effective communication at working levels. On occasion, unions preferred to escalate problem resolution without providing managers the opportunity to address the issue. The hospital continues to work on the principle that problem resolution and decision making take place as close to the source of the issue as possible.

Member Capability

The domain of member capability addresses the knowledge, skills, and commitments of individuals within the organization. Where the hospital's partnerships were concerned, the matter of people's understanding of and capability in decision making became a challenge. This important understanding related to the responsibility and authority for decision making was alluded to earlier. It was important that all those involved in collaborative partnerships understood their respective roles. Were they advisory to the decision, responsible for the development and choice of alternatives, or was the administrative structure responsible for the decision? Any of these alternatives was appropriate, but the parameters of the process must be clearly understood from the outset of consideration of each issue.

Continuing Collaboration

Work in all three domains remains a challenge for the hospital in the creation of successful relationships with partners. The commitment to effective collaboration continues to be an important principle in the total quality management journey.

The examples of partnerships and the keys to success as described in the previous section reinforce the point that partnerships are an important way of doing business in today's world. The ability of organizations to succeed and indeed prosper is influenced greatly by their ability to forge positive and productive relationships with their key stakeholders. Partnerships are essential for organizational transformation and indeed for transformation of the system overall. These partnerships need to be based on the assumption that all parties have something to gain in the partnership—something that could not be achieved without it—and that such gains will not be achieved at the expense of one of the partners.

References

Krackhardt, D. "The Strength of Strong Ties: The Importance of Philos in Organizations." In N. Nohria and R. G. Eccles (eds.), *Networks and Organizations: Structure, Form and Action*. Boston: Harvard Business School Press, 1992.

McClellan, S. Personal correspondence. August 24, 1993.

Schurman, D., and Langlois, W. "Kodak Canada Inc. and University of Alberta Hospitals: Opportunities for Health Care in Canada." *Partners*. Canadian Health Development Foundation. Toronto: June 1993 (Vol. 2), pp. 2–4.

University of Alberta Hospitals. *Management Statement*. Edmonton: University of Alberta Hospitals, 1993.

Part Three

Preparing for the Future

As total quality management and the associated principles were implemented in the University of Alberta Hospital, many initiatives were undertaken in an effort to transform the organization and to move it toward the vision articulated by the senior executive team. Part Two of this book described many of those initiatives.

If one were to ask organizational members whether the organization has actually changed, however, the responses undoubtedly be varied. The hospital was four years into the quality journey when this book was written. It is recognized that such a transformation takes as many as ten years to be truly pervasive. For this reason, reality checks, minor course corrections, and consistent evaluation in light of broader contextual changes must be part of the ongoing activity associated with the implementation of total quality management.

Part Three focuses on these reality checks and anticipates the impact health care reform and system change will have on the organization. Chapter Eleven is, in essence, a dialogue with the senior executive team. On one occasion the members of the team took the opportunity to revisit the principles associated with total quality management in the hospital in an attempt to assess "how are things going?" and "are adjustments/changes required?" Chapter Eleven provides insight into their assessment.

Chapter Twelve addresses challenges: those encountered during the implementation of total quality management and those anticipated as health care reform and transformation of the system occur. It concludes with reflection on total quality management as the philosophy through which to confront the challenges.

Chapter Eleven

Reflecting on Our Principles

Donald P. Schurman

The ability of an organization to continually develop and transform while responding to shifts within the external and internal environments rests with its ability to continually learn as changes are implemented and new understandings are achieved. It is the perception of the executive team at the University of Alberta Hospital that the continued adeptness of the organization to be proactive and to constructively transform as the health care system is experiencing challenge and constraint is, to a large extent, influenced by the capacity of organizational members to move toward the hospital's vision.

The executive team at the University of Alberta Hospital has been committed to the regular review of transformation in the organization within the Organization Capability Development Framework and with respect to the management principles defined and illustrated in Chapters Four to Ten. Additionally, the team is committed to regular assessment of its effectiveness—both individually and collectively—and to continually identifying and implementing processes and concepts that contribute to the organizational transformation initiative within the hospital.

On one occasion, the members of the executive team set aside time to reflect on the management principles as they had been initially articulated and, from their perspective, to assess their reality in practice—the extent to which the organization was succeeding in demonstrating each principle. Additionally, the team evaluated whether each principle clearly conveyed the intent and understanding that had emerged within the organization.

This chapter is an account of that dialogue among the executive team, members of which are also the authors of this book. Included were Donald P. Schurman, President and Chief Executive Officer; Heather A. Andrews, Vice President (Patient Services); Lynn M. Cook, Vice President (Corporate Development); Janet M. Davidson, Vice President (Patient Services); Eric W. Taylor, Vice President (Corporate Support); and Ronald H. Wensel, Vice President (Patient Services). Much of the content is presented in interview format in an attempt to provide the reader with a clear picture of the assessment of organizational transformation at one particular moment. The order in which the principles are presented is altered from that in Part Two of this book, but it reflects the order in which the principles are identified in the hospital's management statement (University of Alberta Hospitals, 1993).

A Dialogue with the Executive Team

The intent of the dialogue was to revisit the management principles as they had been developed by the executive team. Although the principles had existed within the organization for several years, there had been no formal document clearly stating them for members of the organization until one year prior to this discussion. The executive team was engaged in an assessment of whether and how the principles were actually becoming a reality within the organization. As each of the six principles is identified in the following section, the impressions and evaluations of the executive team members are provided.

Customer Satisfaction

> *Customer Satisfaction:* The fundamental reason for this or any enterprise is the satisfaction of our principal external stakeholder—the patient. All resources—time, human energy, technology, and money—should be allocated to this end (University of Alberta Hospitals, 1993, p. 3).

Schurman: Let's spend some time examining our management principles to see if they require amendment, the first one being *customer satisfaction.* Do we still agree with this principle?

Andrews: How can you argue against that? It's like "motherhood and apple pie."

Schurman: I do have some concerns—not with the statement, but with our practice. For example, when I look at the allocation of the resources in the operating room, I sometimes have the sense that we are driven by the need to allocate O.R. time equitably among our surgeons rather than responding to the needs evident on our waiting lists.

Wensel: That's certainly our history, but we are now making changes to enhance the allocation of time—for example, for procedures such as hip replacement and some gynecological procedures—to reflect community needs. Such decisions do, however, need to be balanced against the educational needs of students and the other requirements of an academic health care center.

Davidson: The recent decision regarding relocation of the neurology unit attempted to address many customers. The unit chosen, while perhaps not optimal for the patients, represented a compromise that also attempted to satisfy the education and research interests of the neurology program.

Cook: And if you think about satisfaction for the patient, the care we deliver today satisfies the patient today, but research and education really are designed to satisfy a patient or groups of patients sometime in the future. The decision to support research and education commitments is still directed toward patients—our future patients who also are counting on us.

Davidson: A lot of the concern I have centers around the recent discussions about program relocation within the region. The faculty of medicine appears to be taking the position that, somehow, education and research activities are going to be severely jeopardized if they leave this institution. We should continue to argue that we are first and foremost a hospital that is involved in providing care to patients today or potential patients in the future. Admittedly, we have an important role in education and research, but I would argue that the university's principal stakeholders are the students and the researchers, not the patients.

Cook: Our principles don't stand on their own. They guide our actions in the context of our vision and values. If the vision talks about current patients and population health, then that's an elaboration on who our patients are, today and in the future. The problem is, when you start focusing on specific phrases or words, you'll never get a statement that will meet everybody's needs. I tend to think that the way the statement is currently worded captures our intent—the essence of what we mean by "patient."

Schurman: From my position in the organization, I feel comfortable with these words as the starting point for the management principles. Stating that the patient is the ultimate beneficiary of what we do but recognizing that we have to interpret this with some balance will, I believe, continue to provide our organization with the correct focus.

Andrews: It's almost like Senge's (1990, p. 13) hologram illustration. We, as the executive team, have a certain perspective that we have defined here. Each person in the organization, each group of people, has a different perspective that is complementary but is either more specific or more general. Even among us, we probably have little nuances that would embellish for ourselves this idea of customer satisfaction.

Process Management

Process Management: We recognize that we produce results as a function of the processes we have available to us. The principle of process management is predicated upon an understanding that creating a different future or different results involves changing our processes and organizational practices (University of Alberta Hospitals, 1993, p. 3).

Schurman: Our second management principle, *process management*, simply states that we recognize that results are produced as a function of the processes we have available to us and that we must, therefore, change current processes or add new ones if we desire different results.

Andrews: My sense is that we have really not tested this and that the test is coming with the Patient Care Design Project. There have been instances where processes have been studied in a limited way. The benchmarking study of the admitting process still has a way to go. My sense is that this is an exceedingly important principle but the test is yet to come.

Cook: I believe this principle is absolutely true. If we do things the same way while expecting different results, change and transformation are not going to happen. It's my assessment that we are much better at this at the level of small, individual processes than at the level of big systems. In many organizations, the executive team expects people in the organization to display discipline around process management through the use of the tools and techniques of quality improvement but, when it comes time to do "big work" on behalf of the organization, we don't do it with the same amount of discipline. I would be interested in approaching the redesign of the strategic planning process with more discipline than we have had in the past.

Schurman: What you're talking about is our new understanding of the difference between material processes, people processes, information processes, and what are called the strategic business processes of the organization—for example, our Patient Care Design Project and our planning process. These major processes can also benefit from quality improvement process redesign.

Davidson: It strikes me that we were slightly naive when we included this principle. However, I fundamentally believe that this is the way we need to understand how organizations work. I don't think we initially had as much of an appreciation for what that meant as we do now, and it really comes home through the Patient Care Design Project. This effort involves major system redesign, and our staff are demonstrating significant understanding in knowing how the organization works through processes.

Schurman: When I first reviewed these principles, I didn't think any changes were necessary. As I listen to the dialogue, I wonder if that's correct. What I hear being discussed is the difference between first-order change and second-order change (initially described by Walzlawick, Weakland, and Fisch, 1974). First-order change is continuous improvement while second-order change is fundamental restructuring, like our Patient Care Design Project. There is growing recognition that second order change is what is required to improve organizational performance. Berwick (1993, p. 3) views second-order change as the essence of the quality management process or quality improvement. What is often missing, it seems to me, is an understanding that any change requires new learning. You have to learn something about your processes, change the context in which you work, or acquire new skills or knowledge in order to bring about real change.

Davidson: There is also an issue around personal change being required prior to achieving organizational change.

Schurman: That is a good point. This is a third dimension now being increasingly discussed in the literature—the need for personal change by everyone prior to being able to realize significant organizational improvement.

Taylor: This may be too philosophical. . . . The great innovations, the great creativity of the world does not come by focusing on yesterday's data, yesterday's mistakes, yesterday's processes. It comes from having a vision of trying to create something that has not been created before—you don't have any measurements. The measurement thing can be a trap. A focus on measurement may lock you into first-order change when both first-order and second-order change are necessary.

Schurman: It would seem that three adjustments are required in this management principle: reference to both first- and second-order change is required; process improvement is contingent on learning in an organization; and in order to get organizational change, you have to start with personal change.

Measurable, Observable Results

> *Measurable, Observable Results*: Management effectiveness is dependent on a disciplined focus on measurable, observable outcomes. This is essential if we are to have the feedback we need to intervene skillfully in the design and management of effective processes (University of Alberta Hospitals, 1993, p. 3).

Schurman: Material recently published by Senge (Kofman and Senge, 1993, p. 10) has created some personal uneasiness around this issue. Senge suggests that focusing on measurable, observable results may force you into a short-term time frame. True learning can only take place over a longer time period, and to concentrate too much on trying to get immediate results limits your ability to truly become a learning organization. Senge says there really has to be balance between the measurable, short-term issues and recognizing that some of the interventions you make have a much longer time period for changes to be realized.

Cook: But this principle doesn't say anything about time. If we change the way we do strategic planning, I would hope that we would be able to see something different happening. We should be able to make some observations around the time it takes us to define a plan or the amount of rework that is required. This doesn't speak to time; it just says that management effectiveness and, in fact, learning are dependent on measurable or observable outcomes that are different from what we had before.

Andrews: I believe that measurement is highly important in certain aspects of what we do. But there are other areas that cause me concern with respect to measurement. For example, the data that have been used in some centers involved in patient care redesign to make determinations about targets have been viewed as meaningless by some of the staff of those institutions.

Cook: Is there a possibility that, within an organization that has fully implemented total quality management, data integrity is not an issue? Perhaps their data processes are so sound, they are beyond question.

Andrews: Another concern is the comparability of the data. I believe we use a lot of data that are comparing apples and oranges. To get the real facts underlying the data is often a real challenge. But if the data reflect quality measures from the outset and you are assured that they are comparable, then it would be comfortable to use that data for decision making.

Taylor: There are lots of traps in data. Some people use comparative data to justify the status quo as opposed to looking for opportunities. A focus on continual improvement would suggest that you constantly improve your performance. Therefore, your indicator measurements should be improving regardless of how good or bad the comparative data may look.

Schurman: Our statement is not in conflict with that point of view. I also note that you can look at observable events rather than just data. It seems to me that the principle speaks to demonstrated improvement, which is our responsibility.

Collaboration, Not Consensus

Collaboration, Not Consensus: We believe that all coordination occurs in our relationships with one another, and so it follows that we can only be truly effective in collaboration with those involved, whether on a project, on a team, or on an organizationwide basis. Collaborating means listening to and, if appropriate, acting on the concerns and contributions of others in the course of doing our jobs. It does not mean consensus or universal agreement. Rather, collaboration means involvement and inclusion of others in the design and coordination of work (University of Alberta Hospitals, 1993, p. 3).

Taylor: I believe this is an obvious statement, but it's a question of whether it actually plays itself out in day-to-day activity and whether it should. Some planning discussions now under way are criticized because they are not open and consultative. Perhaps it's not appropriate that they be open.

Davidson: From my point of view, I think that this is one of the more difficult principles that we have. It is my assessment that the organization still seems to want to strive for consensus. Yet true consensus may well result in suboptimal decisions.

Cook: I remember talking about this principle with regard to our organizational restructuring. People were saying, "You did not consult with us." This principle doesn't necessarily mean that, if I'm going to take action today, I have to talk to you today. It means that, at some point, I need to have had some input from you about what you think, what you would recommend.

Schurman: That's exactly it. The last sentence of the statement is significant: "Rather, collaboration means involvement and inclusion of others in the design and coordination. . . ." The word *inclusion* provides an opening for having discussions that involve people without their presence but being concerned for their point of view. Individuals may not be in the room at the time, but you still take their concerns into account as you make decisions.

Taylor: I believe there's a temporal factor here. In some cases you have to act and then include others. There may be situations where a decision model not involving a lot of constituent democracy is appropriate.

Andrews: It is my assessment that this definitely has been an area of confusion. There are people within the organization that believe that involvement in decision making means that everybody will have an opportunity to be involved in every decision. As we tried to develop the governance model, there was a lot of work being done on the decisions into which people would and should have input. The "levels of authority" concept (Cox and Miller, 1991, p. 19) is another parameter of all of this. When you are asking people for their involvement, are you asking for their input, asking them to suggest alternatives, or are you asking them to do the whole thing? The bottom line is that people within the organizational structure have a responsibility for certain aspects of what needs to be done, and we need to seek clarity on the issue.

Davidson: The statement "it does not mean consensus or universal agreement" should perhaps be supplemented by another statement that says, "nor does it mean involvement of everyone in every decision." Rather, collaboration means involvement and inclusion of others in the design and coordination of work.

Taylor: I think that is where collaboration rubs against empowerment and accountability. If people know that a decision is theirs to make, they are going to be empowered. It is their responsibility, and they are accountable. Then, they must be prepared to take action rather than delay the action by going through a process of surveying the world at large.

Schurman: I know what you are saying. However, if freedom not to be collaborative is given to our hard-line/traditional managers, they will take it—and perhaps with a vengeance. We do want people to involve their staff; yet I understand what you are saying. How do we get the balance?

Cook: Now we are talking about *empowerment,* which is another principle. When we talk about empowerment, I think we need to say something about "role." Empowerment is confusing to many. Does it mean I am involved in every decision? Does it mean I make every decision? Empowerment has to be defined within the roles that people have within the organization. Getting back to collaboration, if we believe it is an important principle, collaboration really means making sure that others who are impacted by a decision have some opportunity to provide information and be consulted—but not necessarily from a temporal view or at the time the decision is being made. It may be that consultation takes place in some other way.

Empowerment

Empowerment: As a principle, empowerment is defined as having (or having access to) what is needed for fulfilling our commitments. Most of us recognize that we always have much more power (capacity for action) than we are using at any given time (University of Alberta Hospitals, 1993, p. 4).

Wensel: It seems to me that empowerment is related to an individual's role, as was suggested. Empowerment means having the power necessary to fulfill our commitments, and commitments are generally related to the role of an individual. If one's role can be defined, so can empowerment. There may be individuals who have a commitment far beyond their role. Then empowerment becomes an issue.

Cook: I know there is a lot of confusion about empowerment because some people feel that if they are empowered, they can do whatever they feel needs to be done.

Davidson: Yes, that's a good point. Empowerment means that you are empowered to make the decisions that are within your role, but it does not extend beyond that for you to do whatever you want.

Andrews: Perhaps the first sentence could be changed to read, "the commitments within your defined role."

Cook: For those who want to work on activities beyond their defined role, they can do so through various teams and committees that are suitably empowered.

Andrews: Empowerment is very much an attitude, too. I heard someone speak about empowerment, saying that it is nothing you can give to someone—I can't make you "empowered." A person has to assume an attitude of being empowered. Your behaviors, then, enable you to have access to what you need to be able to perform your role.

Cook: It is important to understand that, at the individual level, power is related to a person's role and his or her ability to fulfill that role. Each person needs his or her own understanding of the context, infrastructure, and member capability associated with his or her role—the hologram again. This will result in empowered people in an empowered organization. Now that would be an empowered organization! That reinforces the importance of a clearly articulated organizational role—organizational participants depend on it, in turn, to define their roles.

Accountability/Teamwork

Accountability/Teamwork: The principle of accountability suggests that no one individual is ever capable of knowing enough or being sufficient to control complex organizational processes. It is therefore crucial that we be able to count on one another, recognizing our different roles and that we are all in this together. Our notion of accountability is "count-on-ability." We must hold people accountable for what we are counting on them to do (University of Alberta Hospitals, 1993, p. 4).

Schurman: There is something missing from this principle. I believe we are sending out inconsistent messages and we must clarify our intentions.

Andrews: I think the first sentence is very important, but maybe it is the principle of *teamwork* that we are talking about rather than *accountability*.

Davidson: We may have made a mistake in grouping those two together because I don't think accountability and teamwork are the same.

Andrews: But based on the definition of accountability—suggesting that no one person can be expected to know everything about the organization—it demands that one depend on the team.

Davidson: Well, I think that it would be better to call it "accountability and teamwork" rather than "accountability/ teamwork," so that we understand that if you are going to be accountable, you have got to work with a team. Would that work for you, Don?

Taylor: What about the concept of role again? A clearly defined role helps people define what they are accountable for.

Schurman: The recommendation regarding changing the title of this principle to "accountability and teamwork" is helpful. It places the words of this principle in their proper context.

Andrews: Another perspective that has been helpful in understanding accountability has been developed by Cox and Miller (1991, p. 19). They stress the importance of having a common understanding of responsibility, authority, and accountability and that each element must exist in combination with the others. Responsibility is ownership plus impact and must be given and accepted. This, combined with authority (the right to act in areas of responsibility) and accountability (retrospective evaluation), produces truly effective decentralized decision making. This, to me, ties in nicely with the idea that we count on people to fulfill certain roles in the organization.

Effective Relationships

Effective Relationships: Effective relationships are essential to accomplishing anything together and to achieving results in a manner in which people experience as empowering (University of Alberta Hospitals, 1993, p. 4).

Schurman: Lastly we should review the principle of *effective relationships* and the dialogue ground rules that guide our work with others. The first ground rule is "listen generously."

Listen Generously: This means learning to listen to the contribution and commitment of the other person and suspending assessments, judgments, and opinions about what he or she is saying. This does not mean that we agree or disagree with what is being said, but that we are committed to the legitimacy and value of the view (University of Alberta Hospitals, 1993, p. 4).

Cook: I think that these ground rules give our management principles a lot of power. Many organizations talk about accountability and process management and using the tools and techniques of quality improvement. But I have seen very few other organizations' management principles include ground rules for how people work together—specifically and explicitly outlined. If there is a shortcoming, it may be that we don't highlight the Basic Action Workflow Process (see Chapter Four) and the idea of requests, offers, and commitments as a way of coordinating action. We jump right into these dialogue ground rules. Should we enhance this by referring to the process involved in any interaction?

Andrews: As much as we acknowledge the importance of generous listening, it is something with which I continue to be challenged. The understanding of the process underlying effective relationships has helped a lot and I agree with you; we should add a statement conveying that idea.

Talk Straight: This means speaking honestly in a way that forwards the action as opposed to reacting to or attacking what is being said. This includes learning to make clear and direct requests (University of Alberta Hospitals, 1993, p. 4).

Schurman: The most significant challenge here is to speak straight in a way that forwards the action. We have an ability to speak straight, but sometimes it has the impact of slowing progress rather than advancing it. In some of our recent meetings with the unions, our relationships may actually have deteriorated. In some of those cases, we may not have listened generously, and when we spoke straight, we did so in a way that was not constructive.

Davidson: I think we need to be much more rigorous about using these ground rules to guide our actions. We must reaffirm the purpose of our executive team meetings as a time to review our work as a group and to assess our performance against the ground rules for dialogue to see how we could be more effective. We can and must be more rigorous about our commitment to these.

Schurman: Part of the problem in making this live, however, is related to a mutual understanding of these principles and ground rules. I believe it is easier to speak straight within our executive team than it is to do so with outside individuals since they may be speaking a different language. For example, we appreciate that a negative assessment is one of the few ways we have to create a dialogue that will result in improved performance, yet others become immediately defensive if a negative assessment is provided. We have to recognize the need for this ongoing development in our staff and others.

Be For Each Other. This means believing in and committing ourselves to the premise that we are all in this together and that no one individual can win at the expense of another. This is the basis for trust and for making it safe for each other to take risks without fear of censure or of being undermined by one's colleagues (University of Alberta Hospitals, 1993, p. 4).

Schurman: This is a challenging principle, given the risks and the possibility of being undermined as regional program transfers are being considered. It is not clear who is supportive and who is opposed.

Cook: We talk about how critical these ground rules are for effective relationships within teams, but often, even if you consider executive teams, it does not necessarily mean that these are practiced. It has taken us a lot of time and effort to get to the stage where we feel any one of us can go away on vacation and feel supported in our area in the executive team when we are gone. When we think about being part of this other team—the regional team—we have to recognize that that group has not done any developmental work and may not have a relationship sufficient for the task at hand. Our executive team has been committed to making this happen within our team.

Davidson: Based on the principle of collaboration, I have faith in what you are doing with respect to regional planning, Don [Schurman]. Even though there is a chance that, in a year from now, our organizational and individual roles may be completely different, I do believe that the attempts to establish a new governance system for health care in the region is appropriate and important and consistent with this principle.

Taylor: Returning to our organization, I sense that there is still a great deal of competitiveness within the organization. The change in organizational structure (see Chapter Six) may, in fact, encourage some of that competitiveness. For some situations, I think you see it exhibited where people are trying to win at the expense of others. For example, our budget discussions continue to be competitive in nature.

Schurman: Peter Senge is working with a group of organizations trying to really understand how to create learning organizations. He notes, in a recent article (Kofman and Senge, 1993, p. 7), three general problems in our society: (1) fragmentation—we still do not understand systems thinking, (2) reactiveness—we still tend to react to things more than being driven by a vision of the future, and (3) competitiveness—he notes there are some excellent aspects of competition but also that it is apparent in our society that the way it often shows up is counterproductive.

This whole issue of competitiveness is one that is a challenge to manage. Some aspects are good, but it must be contained.

Taylor: There is a cultural bias toward competitiveness because of the way we have been raised. Perhaps we should just recognize that it exists and try and go with the flow and use it in a constructive way as opposed to trying to fight something that could be a good thing.

Andrews: We must remember that we have developed particular roles for staff that are focused on particular areas of service. We expect them to intervene on behalf of their areas. As they focus on the benefits for their particular responsibilities, there is a perception of competition when perhaps they are simply fulfilling the expectations we have of them.

Cook: Part of the problem may be that newly developed roles have been assigned to a recently restructured leadership group—the people who are responsible for the high-level design and implementation of systems within the organization to cause it to be more effective. Work on relationships within that group is beginning. The executive team will be required to assess capability gaps in that group now and encourage the members together to do the kinds of things we do together as an executive team to create effective relationships, to understand that whatever they do to be successful cannot be at the expense of somebody else's success.

Davidson: I suppose one could argue that there is healthy competition—competition based on performance outcome. With respect to "being for each other," perhaps we should expect more from management staff regarding the sharing of new learning on a continuing basis.

Honor One Another's Commitments. This means respecting one anothers' commitments, including your own (University of Alberta Hospitals, 1993, p. 5).

Davidson: The greatest challenge is in understanding the commitments of others.

Schurman: This ground rule comes alive when we begin to recognize that the actions of every individual are motivated by his or her commitments. Recognizing this reality, this challenges each of us to look at commitments when conflict is noted. In that regard, this ground rule is powerful, as it results in a dialogue about commitment and forces breakthrough solutions rather than forcing one party to abandon his or her commitment.

Cook: Another important understanding relates to what a commitment is in terms of the basic action workflow process. In that model, a commitment is an "offer" or "promise." In certain circumstances it may be necessary to revisit commitments, particularly if circumstances arise that interfere with their achievement. There may or may not be consequences associated with the alteration or retraction of commitments.

Acknowledge and Appreciate One Another. This means that each member of the team commits to continuously acknowledge and appreciate the contributions of others and the team itself, even when things do not work out. It also means requesting and receiving acknowledgment from others if it is missing for you (University of Alberta Hospitals, 1993, p. 5).

Schurman: The second component, namely seeking acknowledgment, is not well done. And even though it may look self-serving, the challenging environment requires peer group recognition. It is an important ground rule that is clear in its intention. A commitment to use this ground rule is necessary from all.

Cook: The importance of this ground rule was emphasized by our management staff in their description of being truly compensated—acknowledgment and appreciation were high on the list of factors.

Be Concerned for Inclusion: This means asking the question, "Who else should be included in or has a stake in what we are talking about?" (University of Alberta Hospitals, 1993, p. 5).

Taylor: The only dilemma is that many people have the idea that they have to be involved in everything all the time. There should be acceptance that everyone does not have to be there all the time in order to thrive.

Davidson: One of the interesting dimensions of this statement is the phrase "who have a stake in what we are talking about." It helps determine who should be involved in particular issues.

Schurman: I find this statement empowering since it does not tell me that everyone has to be there but, rather, demands that an individual think about who is affected and acknowledge and represent the fact that they may have a different point of view even if they are not present. The fact that there are some who feel they need to be personally involved is one that continues to frustrate me. All of us could be in three or four places at any time. We have to begin to feel confident that others will represent our point of view when we are not present.

Davidson: I think that we have not done as good a job with this. While we, the executive team, are trying to divest ourselves of responsibility in things that we do not believe we need to be involved in, there are still many staff who feel that a vice president should be involved in all decisions to make sure that they are "on side."

Taylor: I agree. In some cases I think it is the idea that unless the vice president is there and says something or makes a decision, the result is not going to fly. It may be in a mind-set of others that I have to be there. On the other hand, is there something that I am doing that continues to encourage this—that says that they really do have to bring me in? So again, there is a two-way street here. Because, if staff really get signals that say I have to be there every time something goes on, then clearly, they are going to continue to ask.

Cook: One of the vehicles that will help us with this is the performance management system. When we are talking about competencies and the level at which we expect executive and management to perform the various competencies, we should see increased clarification of authority, accountability, responsibility, and performance.

Be Concerned for Alignment: This means participating in every conversation with a commitment to build alignment. Alignment does not mean consensus or universal agreement. It means that everyone is either "committed to" or "able to support" the commitments of others. No one is committed against the direction in which we are moving (University of Alberta Hospitals, 1993, p. 5).

Andrews: I think something that has been a concern in the past actually involves the last two ground rules—acknowledging that, at all times, inclusion may not be appropriate or necessary, but then, the implication that exclusion has for alignment. We have had occasions where, in team discussions, all of us have not been present. Then, at a point down the road, we find that we are not all aligned.

Schurman: These ground rules would be helpful at regional planning with the difficult issues that we are facing. Yet one individual has been successful in keeping the group from discussions involving his organization because he has purposely stayed away. Nor is he aligned with what the members are trying to accomplish, and this has worked to his advantage.

Andrews: This points out the importance of these ground rules in relation to an effective organization because, if any of them is missing as an ingredient, then the effectiveness is not there.

Lessons Learned

This chapter has presented a dialogue among the executive team of the University of Alberta Hospital focused on the management principles as set forth in the philosophy associated with the organization's commitment to total quality management. As was evident in the dialogue, the principles as they were initially developed remain sound. A few specific amendments were inserted to clarify the intent of the principles for the organization.

The discussion surrounding the principles is of critical importance in the highly volatile and constantly changing context of the health care system. By continually reviewing the organization's status in relation to the preferred future, the principles guide the action of the team, equipping it to lead the organization in its ongoing transformation.

Toward the end of the dialogue, it became evident that new and fundamental issues beyond the walls of the organization are emerging in the health care system and commanding the attention of the executive team. Within the provincial health care arena, significant and broader changes are becoming reality. This turbulent world requires completely new and innovative responses. Working at the margins will not yield significant results.

References

Berwick, D. "Improving Community Health Status." *Quality Connection*, 1993, 2(3), 2–3.

Cox, S., and Miller, D. *Leaders Empower Staff*. Minneapolis, Minn.: Creative Nursing Management, 1991.

Hammer, M., and Champy, J. *Reengineering the Corporation: A Manifesto for Business Revolution*. New York: HarperCollins, 1993.

Kofman, F., and Senge, P. M. "Communities of Commitment: The Heart of Learning Organizations." In D. Bohl and F. Luthan (eds.), *Organizational Dynamics*. New York: American Management Association, 1993.

Senge, P. "The Leader's New Work: Building Learning Organizations." *Sloan Management Review*, Fall 1990, pp. 7–23.

University of Alberta Hospitals. *Management Statement*. Edmonton: University
    of Alberta Hospitals, 1993.
Walzlawick, P., Weakland, J., and Fisch, R. *Change*. New York: W. W. Norton,
    1974.

Chapter Twelve

Surmounting the Challenges

Donald P. Schurman
Heather A. Andrews

The experience at the University of Alberta Hospital during the implementation of total quality management has contributed significantly to an understanding of the challenges of organizational transformation. The successes and failures addressed in this book are presented with the objective of providing other organizational change agents and leaders the benefit of understanding and insight associated with experience. The challenges addressed in this chapter entail both those that were encountered and those that are anticipated—the aspects of health care reform that nations around the globe are encountering in the 1990s.

This chapter is based primarily on a dialogue among the senior executive team during which they evaluated the process and outcomes/results experienced during the initial years of the transformation. Extensive reference to recent literature contributes to an overview of the fundamental issues and challenges associated with health care reform and its implications for the organization.

Challenges in Retrospect

As one reviews the experiences associated with organizational transformation and the implementation of total quality management at the University of Alberta Hospital, a number of factors emerge that presented particular and complex challenges during the process of change. The three domains of the Organization Capability

Development Framework as described in Chapter Two provide a system for categorizing and analyzing these challenges.

Contextual Challenges

Although the contextual perspective presented in Chapter Two was confined to the context *within* the organization, discussion of context in this chapter takes on a broader perspective to include aspects of the organizational environment beyond the walls of the institution. As Scott (1992, p. 99) notes, "The field of organizational research has for too long excluded consideration of the larger environmental forces that push and constrain the structures and processes characterizing its individual units. To artificially restrict attention to the internal workings of such units is, for most issues, to misunderstand their nature and to misinterpret their operations."

Context was described in Chapter Two as consisting of the components of mission, vision, values, principles, strategies, and objectives. The same components are relevant from the perspective of the system as a whole. Problems and challenges occur when there is dissonance between the system and the organizational context or when the system context is virtually undefined. Such was the case at the University of Alberta Hospital. The most significant challenges developed in relation to other stakeholders in the context of the health care system—government, the other organizations in the region, unions, and the university.

Government. As the University of Alberta Hospital proceeded in its transformation toward a philosophy and practice of total quality management, the provincial government could best be described as an interested bystander. Although there were many attempts to enrol Alberta Health in the philosophy of total quality management or to involve specific representatives in certain initiatives, the opportunity was consistently bypassed. Government representatives, understandably, felt that, since their mandate rested with the entire province, involvement with organization-specific initiatives would prove difficult and might compromise their objectivity from the perspectives of other stakeholders. As a result, government's involvement was remote. However, from a distance, there were indications of interest and encouragement. Several projects associated with the transformation (for example, the nursing governance project) were supported with enabling grants from government.

This limited involvement was a source of much frustration. The government was not committed to the total quality management philosophy, and it became disconcerting for staff to interact with an agency that did not hold similar values or adhere to the same principles as their organization. As hospital employees began to disdain inefficient processes and ineffective internal activities, they still were required to respond to demands from governmental agencies even though they were often viewed as waste, rework, or redundant activity.

Regional Organizations. As the organizational transformation was proceeding, aspects of system reform challenged the process. Discussions at the regional tables involving senior representatives from health care organizations hypothesized about program amalgamation, institutional mergers, and closures of hospitals. Although few would deny the need for such actions, uncertainty and rumors about future possibilities adversely affected the commitment of employees and physicians to total quality management and to the organization, diverted the attention and time of senior staff, and disrupted constancy of purpose and commitment to a unified vision for the organization.

Regional fiscal constraints also posed a challenge for the hospital's implementation of total quality management. As funding was cut, operations were reduced and staff were laid off. The atmosphere of threat and uncertainty appeared to compromise the ability of employees to totally commit to the new philosophy, and the disruption to service delivery caused by the layoff and recall processes dictated in the collective agreements called into question the organizational commitment to the principles of total quality management. For example, employees questioned, "If the organization is truly committed to patient/customer satisfaction, how can the 'bumping' of experienced staff through the layoff process be condoned by the hospital?"

Although it had been the commitment of the executive team to base the organizational transformation on the management principles associated with total quality management rather than the financial imperative, there were several points in the journey at which the team members wondered if financial viability would have provided greater impetus for the transformation than did a principle-based motive. As Donald P. Schurman, president and chief executive officer of the University of Alberta Hospital, stated in a dialogue with the executive team in December 1993,

> I have always wanted to stay away from finances driving our efforts and instead make this a quality issue, recognizing that the dollars would somehow look after themselves. Even if we are excellent at process improvement, however, I have a bit of a concern that, as we put pressure on the dollars, most of the dialogue will be around the restructuring necessary to satisfy the financial agenda. If so, our change efforts will be based less on the management principles and more on the imperative to survive. That does not become a very inspiring vision, but there may be nothing we can do about it.

Unions. The unionized environment in which the University of Alberta Hospital exists presented a particular challenge. As the implementation of total quality management proceeded, many attempts were made to forge effective partnerships with the hospital's four stakeholder unions. The hospital was several years into the transformation process when the reason for ongoing confrontation and relational problems became clear.

The challenge rested with the differing contextual perspectives of the hospital and the various associations. As Janet M. Davidson, Vice President (Patient Services) at the University of Alberta Hospital, points out, ". . . if a union is committed to maintaining the maximum number of individuals it can, and to ensuring that those individuals have all their rights protected by virtue of their collective agreement, its number one objective is not patient care" (dialogue with the executive team, December 6, 1993). For instance, as much as the executive team wanted to involve key union representatives in decision making at the senior level, the decision process in the unions—consultation with members before taking a position—did not permit effective involvement at a table where decisions were to be made at the moment. It also became clear that, because of their mandate, union representatives could not involve themselves in decisions that could adversely affect their members.

As it became apparent that the missions, visions, values, and decision-making processes of the various organizations differed substantially, new ways were sought to effectively relate, communicate, and work together as the transformation proceeded. The forums that proved particularly effective were labor-management liaison committees wherein issues of mutual concern were addressed, hospital directions were communicated, and problems of a general nature were resolved.

The University. As an academic medical center, the University of Alberta Hospital fulfills its triple mission of patient care, teaching, and research in close affiliation with the University of Alberta. The challenges associated with the administration of an academic medical center and the partnership with the university became increasingly apparent as total quality management became a reality.

As Blumenthal and Meyer (1993, p. 1812) describe, "For these centers [academic medical centers] to survive, let alone prosper, their leaders, faculty, and staff members need a clear, unromanticized understanding of the changed environment they face and of the comparative advantages and disadvantages that their institutions bring to these new situations." The transformation under way at the University of Alberta Hospital was viewed as the approach to tackle these issues.

Since the hospital is operated as an entirely separate organization from the University of Alberta, with a distinct board and administrative structure, the organizational transformation to total quality management at the hospital was additionally complicated, given the shared obligation of the hospital and the university. Most medical staff have joint appointments and, therefore, two organizations to whom they are responsible. Indeed, the most senior medical administrators—department chairs—are recruited and appointed jointly by the university and the hospital and have significant obligations to both parties. The jurisdictional lines between the two organizations often blur, making alignment critically important to minimize conflict. The partnership between the two organizations had to be made meaningful and effective if they were to forcefully address the challenge.

The hospital traditionally focused its partnership with the university primarily on the faculty of medicine, a perspective that may have compromised the synergy of a possible relationship with the university as a whole. Throughout the implementation of total quality management, the university and the faculty of medicine have remained on the sidelines.

The faculties with which the hospital has the closest linkages were viewed within the hospital as remote and unrealistic with significant philosophical differences, particularly with respect to the principles of total quality management as they were articulated for the hospital. As Heather A. Andrews, Vice President (Patient Services) at the University of Alberta Hospital points out, "This may be due to the academic independence that universities encourage, but it is manifest by faculty members making judgments about what is happening in the practice setting, not based on any exploration about the reasons or any attempt to understand why certain actions have been taken. This then interferes with their future ability to work with the organization" (dialogue with the executive team, December 6, 1993). As Eric W. Taylor, Vice President (Corporate Support) at the University of Alberta Hospital, describes, "It is impossible for educational institutions to keep up to date with everything that is going on in every industry and create a standard product for everybody. What academic institutions have to do is provide sufficient capability for graduates to gain employment, and then become more involved in helping upgrade on a continuous basis the skills of graduates" (dialogue with the executive team, December 6, 1993). Andrews further observes, "I perceive a difference in philosophical perspectives. Academics believe that educational institutions inform practice. Those in the field believe that practice should inform education. Reality is probably somewhere in the middle."

Much work remains in the creation of an effective and powerful partnership between the two organizations. It is anticipated that two major joint undertakings will assist: (1) the involvement of departmental chairs and divisional directors in the articulation of a strategic operating vision for the hospital and (2) the participation of faculty members in the activities associated with the Patient Care Design Project. By involving the university in addressing major challenges, it is anticipated that the contextual dissonance between the organizations will move toward effective alignment.

Infrastructure Challenges

The challenges associated with the domain of infrastructure pertain to the systems, processes, and procedures—technical, relational, and developmental—existing within the organization.

Technical Issues. From the technical perspective, the hospital has not yet achieved an effective focus on the management of key processes. Although key processes in the organization were identified and assigned to executive members as major responsibilities, they have not yet become a meaningful aspect of the hospital's operation. It is anticipated that, as the Patient Care Design Project comes to fruition, the focus on the management of key processes will play a more significant role in the organization's structure and operation.

A technical issue that became a challenge as the implementation of total quality management proceeded pertained to the management of information within the hospital. There was significant mistrust of the accuracy and inclusiveness of data available through the information systems in the organization. This compromised the employees' willingness to base their actions on the data available to them and resulted in much energy being devoted to disclaiming the validity of the data rather than moving toward creating the future.

Again, the Patient Care Design Project is expected to address some of these issues. Information management systems will be required to respond to the needs identified within patient care processes and patient support processes, where the pattern in the past had been the creation of systems to which the entire organization responded.

Relational Issues. From the relational point of view, the size and complexity of the organization posed a challenge in the implementation of total quality management and the associated transformation of the organization. With a staff of over five thousand people, an autonomous and independent medical staff, and an around-the-clock operation, the ability to ensure an informed work force committed to the change was a pervasive challenge.

Another complicating factor was the relationship of medical resident staff to the hospital. These doctors were not "on staff" and their time with the organization was limited, yet their practice greatly influenced the efficiency and effectiveness of the delivery of care within the hospital. In addition, their loyalty and commitment rested primarily with their educational program rather than with the hospital. The process of transformation did not effectively attend to the involvement or role of that group of practitioners.

Some ideas were put forward to assist with this challenge in the longer term. It was suggested that quality improvement be included as part of the undergraduate curriculum so that new practitioners would be prepared to enter practice with an understanding of the quality improvement philosophy and process. Elective courses for residents in quality management have proven effective in some jurisdictions as well. As medical staff become committed to quality management, they will provide more effective role models for the residents and undergraduates in the system as well.

The medical staff also presented a challenge in the transformation of the organization. As independent and autonomous practitioners, they traditionally have had limited accountability to the organization yet significant impact on resource consumption. The challenge has been to enrol the medical staff in a timely fashion. As Ronald H. Wensel, Vice President (Patient Services) at the University of Alberta Hospital, observes, "The medical staff are aware of the change and the need for change, but we are perhaps only about a quarter of the way on the journey to getting medical staff involved. There are some growing examples of success. I think it is fortunate that this economic environment is driving some of the change because I believe there will be much greater commitment from medical staff due to the economic imperative" (dialogue with the executive team, December 6, 1993).

Part of the problem complicating the situation pertained to the different recognition and reward structures associated with academic medicine. Where the university highly values research and publications, the hospital, particularly in an environment of total quality, values tangible demonstration of the associated principles and practice. Meaningful integration of the two systems would greatly enhance the relationship of medical staff and the hospital.

As well, the hospital must find ways of enhancing recognition and the profile of medical staff who are demonstrating the principles and processes of total quality management.

Developmental Issues. The developmental aspect of the infra-structure is perhaps the most challenging because it is fundamentally related to the building of a learning organization. Little is known regarding the specific requirements for building systems to continuously enhance the capabilities of staff members. Organizational improvement is, however, dependent on individual, personal change. This suggests that there should be disciplined systems of learning that incorporate new knowledge and skill into practice.

Significant efforts now underway by leaders like Kofman and Senge (1993) may result in breakthroughs in understanding the dynamics of building more effective organizations.

Capability Development Challenges

Capability development pertains to the knowledge, skills, and commitments of the members and the organization. The relationship between the medical staff within the hospital posed a significant challenge in this domain as well. The independent practice of the medical staff and the time-limited involvement of the resident staff meant that these people did not avail themselves of the developmental opportunities that were provided for other staff. By the time it was recognized that a different mechanism for enroling the medical staff was required, the transformation to total quality management was already well along. Perhaps greater and faster success with medical staff could have been achieved if they had been enroled earlier in the change. However, as Wensel observes, perhaps the significance of the financial imperative has contributed in the longer term to a growing commitment to quality improvement by physicians (dialogue with the executive team, December 6, 1993).

Middle management within the hospital also posed a challenge. With the focus on the enrolment and development of front-line staff and the perceived threat that empowerment and decentralization of decision making posed for middle management, it became evident that this group was inhibiting the effectiveness of the change, particularly as assessed by the union personnel. There was a growing understanding that the philosophy and practice of total quality management was not consistent throughout the organization at the middle management levels. It was anticipated that the implementation of the performance management system as described in Chapter Eight would address this issue.

These and other instances of lack of commitment to the principles and practice of total quality management compromised and delayed the success and progress of organizational transformation. As Kofman and Senge (1993, p. 5) observe, "moving forward is an exercise in personal commitment and community building. . . . Without communities of people genuinely committed, there is no real chance of going forward."

As the dependency of organizational transformation on personal or individual transformation became clear, the importance of the pursuit of continuous learning was apparent— in particular, the challenge to the senior executive members to continually search for new and better ways of leading the organization. As a result, the team participated in regular development activities, including work on an ongoing basis with a coach, Jim Selman (coauthor of Chapter Four). This activity markedly enhanced both individual capabilities and the ability of the group to function as a team in leading the organization.

Opportunities for capability development that were particularly effective for staff included educational opportunities offered by the hospital, organizational support for members to attend conferences and forums outside the organization, and the expertise of the diverse individuals who were brought into the organization to provide special training. The eclectic approach of the executive team in applying the beneficial and complementary aspects of various approaches to and frameworks of total quality management and organizational transformation enabled the organization to capture the best ideas being forwarded by the most progressive contemporary thinkers and practitioners.

Also related to capability development were the advantages associated with having a consistent and cohesive executive team. This, throughout the implementation of total quality management, provided constancy of senior vision and philosophy with an unwavering commitment to leading the organization through the required change.

As the challenges were identified and addressed, some were dealt with successfully, others less so. Prior knowledge of the problems that tend to emerge undoubtedly would have influenced the manner in which the organizational transformation was orchestrated. The opportunity to apply this learning may present itself at another level of transformation—the system as a whole.

Upcoming Challenges: Health Care Reform

The hospital's experiences—what has worked well within the organization and the challenges that have been encountered and addressed—are now becoming relevant at the level of the system as a whole. It is no longer possible for an organization to be insular in its activities and service to its customers. Consideration now turns to the reform facing the health care system and the potential of total quality management to provide the vehicle to address the reformation.

At the heart of the call for fundamental reform are perspectives such as those forwarded by Gaylin (1993) and McKnight (1994). Gaylin, a physician, in an essay entitled "Faulty Diagnosis: Why Clinton's Health-care Plan Won't Cure What Ails Us," claims, "The paradox of our current situation . . . is that unless we address such basic, almost existential questions, we stand little chance of solving our nation's health-care crisis." (1993, p. 57). He argues that there are basic forces driving rising health care costs: "our unbridled appetite for health care and our continuing expansion of the definition of what constitutes health."

Gaylin (pp. 59–61) identifies four principal causes of escalating health costs: (1) *The increase in morbidity rates due to good medicine*. He claims that "good medicine keeps sick people alive, thereby increasing the number of sick people in the population." (2) *The expanding concept of health*. Conditions that were previously not considered a disease (for example, infertility) now have "treatments" and "cures." (3) *The seduction of technology and the deception of the marketplace models*. "People will pay anything to defend against the possibility of death, all the more so when the money involved doesn't come directly out of their own pockets." (4) *The American character and appetite*. "Americans refuse to believe there are limits—even to life itself." Although Gaylin (p. 62) suggests this attitude differs from that in countries such as Britain and Canada, there are those (the authors) who would claim amazing similarities.

In considering population health, the importance and relevance of the community is becoming increasingly understood. In a lecture to health care personnel, McKnight (1994), director of community affairs at the Center for Urban Affairs and Policy Research in Evanston, Illinois, makes the following assessments: "We [society] have the ability to create crime-making law enforcement agencies, stupid-making educational institutions, and illness-making health care agencies." McKnight believes, as do an increasing number of others, that the determinants of health status are not associated with the number of hospital beds in a region but with the community. He advocates rebuilding the fabric of mutual responsibility of communities, the essence of which he claims has been usurped by the bureaucratic hierarchy. McKnight suggests that there is no future in investing more in medical systems; they cannot deal with the social ills of pollution, poverty, and unhealthy lifestyles. In short, McKnight's thesis is this: systems (such as the health care system) produce goods and services that demand consumers and clients (patients). Through their existence, bureaucratic systems diminish the relevance of the community and its ability to confront social ills through the services it offers; it is a zero-sum game.

As the facets of health care reform have become clearer to the leaders in the system, five major aspects have emerged as pillars that will become foundational to the new system. These "pillars" or major issues relate to the following topics: (1) a systemic perspective of health care, (2) organizational and system redesign, (3) health care evaluation, (4) societal expectations, and (5) system financing. Each of these issues is much broader than one organization's role and activity; the implications associated with each have the potential to create massive change in the health care system as it is currently understood.

Systemic Perspective of Health Care

As organizational leaders are addressing the future of health care and broader social systems, they also are facing fundamental questions about relevance, cost/benefit ratio, and even continuing existence. Such dilemmas extend far beyond the boundaries of one organization and into the system as a whole. Certainly, the need for internal organizational change is mandatory, but the change required from the system perspective must also influence organizational response.

In a recent Alberta Health (1993, p. 7) publication, the place of health care services in the broader social system was addressed: "There is more to good health than health care services, for example, the quality of our physical and social environments. The challenge is to maintain and improve our health and the quality of our health system, as we respond to changing social and economic times." The characteristic fragmentation of the system and the resulting suboptimization (improvement of the parts at the expense of the whole) will no longer be tolerated.

Kofman and Senge (1993, p. 7) believe that this fragmentation is one of three fundamental cultural dysfunctions, along with competition and reactiveness: "We continually fragment problems into pieces; yet the major challenges we face in our organizations and beyond are increasingly systemic." They claim that "fragmentation is the cornerstone of what it means to be a professional. We [physicians, managers, accountants, administrators] fragment complex situations into symptoms, treat the symptoms, and rarely inquire into the deeper causes of problems."

The results of fragmentation within the health care system are the regional problems of today. Throughout North America, for example, constituencies are concluding that there are too many acute care beds. Contrary to the assumption of the past, health status of the population does not vary directly with the number of hospital beds. The same pattern of "overbedding" (40 to 50 percent) evident in Boston (Berwick, 1993, p. 2) is reflected in Alberta and in other parts of Canada.

Berwick (1993, p. 2) differentiates between "local heroism" and "system improvement." He states, "in an organizational context, that idea—the difference between local heroism and systemic improvement—is at the core of the challenge of improvement. The challenge is to connect the parts to the system as a whole; to allow every single element of the system, upon which the outside world depends, to understand its place in the whole and to act together." What is required from the perspective of the health care system is the second-order improvement described by Walzlawick, Weakland, and Fisch (1974) and applied to health care by Berwick (1993, p. 3): we must change the system "instead of making changes within the system."

In the Canadian and particularly the Albertan context, changes toward a systemic perspective will mean changes in governance of institutions. It is anticipated that individual hospital boards will be unified into regional boards responsible for the health services provided to specified communities. The resulting regionalization is expected to lead to the merging of hospitals and to changes in the roles of health care and allied organizations, with alterations in programs and services offered by particular providers. Artificial segregation of health care services will no longer be tolerated as the system of care delivery is unified.

It is the systemic perspective that considers the role of the community in the maintenance of health (see McKnight, 1994). As reform is undertaken, hospitals will forge new ties with the communities they serve and new and more effective linkages will be sought that contribute to and promote population health. The shape of such linkages remains to be seen.

Organizational Redesign

Associated with the issue of a systemic perspective, yet affecting organizations and systems alike, is the notion of redesign, restructuring, or reengineering. Reflective of the second-order change referred to earlier, redesign has the potential to reform organizational processes related to the delivery of care and services to the patients within the health care system, to reform organizational structures as we know them today, and to influence the shaping of the health care system as the reformation proceeds. Byrne (1993, p. 76) advocates, in relation to the traditional hierarchy, "Forget the pyramid. Smash the hierarchy, break the company into its key processes, and create teams from different departments to run them."

Reengineering (used here synonymously with *redesign* and *restructuring*) was defined by Hammer and Champy (1993, p. 46) as "the fundamental rethinking and radical redesign of business processes to achieve dramatic improvement in critical, contemporary measures of performance, such as cost, quality, service, and speed." From the viewpoint of care processes, the University of Alberta Hospital's Patient Care Design Project, as described in Chapter Nine, serves as an example of redesign of the systems associated with the delivery of care and services to the patient.

As Byrne (1993) claims, such reengineering and redesign will also be required of our organizational structures. Peters (1987) advocates a total reconceptualization (revolution) of the management of organizations. Many of his recommendations and solutions reflect the premises of total quality management—focus on customers, empowerment, a new role for management. In addition, he emphasizes fast-paced innovation and the ability to evoke leadership at all levels.

Blackburn and Ridky (1993) describe the evolution of organized enterprise from the division of labor associated with scientific management, to the hierarchical corporation as we know it today, to the information- or knowledge-based organization of the future. Senge (1991) identifies the characteristics of the knowledge-based organization as shared vision, thinking and acting at all levels, systemic thinking (understanding and consideration of interrelationships), and integrative resolution (dialogue and integration of diverse views in decision making). He speculates that organizations will move progressively toward self-directed and self-managed work teams, with management increasingly accountable to staff.

From the systems perspective, creative change versus prescriptive change will be required. New ideas will replace the reinvention of the past. The system, including the professionals, will become accountable to and directed by society rather than the other way around, with society at the mercy of the professionals and the system. The health care system will be held responsible for the evaluation of its offerings.

Health Care Evaluation

The issues raised by Gaylin (1993) and presented earlier in this chapter prompt serious consideration of the benefits of health care as we know it today. As society becomes increasingly aware of these questions, accountability will be demanded of providers.

The third pillar of health care reform pertains to the measurement and evaluation of the outcomes of health care. Nash (1993, p. 396) identifies three aspects of quality for which hospitals will be expected to be accountable: (1) continuous quality improvement, (2) outcomes management, and (3) clinical practice guidelines and standards. O'Leary (1993) suggests that the dimension of quality in health care can be linked with performance and outcomes.

The Joint Commission on Accreditation of Healthcare Organizations (1993, pp. 51–58) identifies nine dimensions of performance: appropriateness, effectiveness, safety, continuity of care, timeliness, efficacy, efficiency, availability, and patient satisfaction. Nelson (1993, p. 371) defines outcomes in terms of "clinical outcomes (mortality, morbidity, complications, symptoms), general health status (physical, emotional, and social functioning), the patient's assessment of the goodness of care (patient satisfaction), and total cost including direct medical cost and indirect social costs." According to O'Leary (1993, p. 487), "Report card day is coming. There is now a social mandate for performance measurement. . . . Almost every reform proposal being introduced at federal and state levels includes a requirement for measuring performance, outcomes, and reporting performance information."

The measurement and evaluation of health care will also have implications for education and research in academic medical centers, according to Blumenthal and Meyer (1993, p. 1813): "The customers of our health care system want . . . its research organizations to generate more knowledge about improving outcomes and the quality of care, and its providers to produce health services with increasing efficiency." It is Blumenthal and Meyer's assessment that, at present, most academic medical centers do not have the resources to accomplish this. The situation could lead to the forging of new relationships with providers, communities, and relevant disciplines. An example of such a relationship is the Healthcare Quality and Outcomes Research Center at the University of Alberta, funded, in part, by the Alberta Heritage Fund for Medical Research. The hospital is pursuing partnership in the initiative as well.

Societal Expectations

The reform required in the health care system will have implications for consumers, professionals, unions, and all other stakeholders. From the perspective of the professionals, roles are expected to change, as are methods of remuneration. Gone are the days when the system was designed around the needs of the professionals. Rather, the needs and expectations of the consumers and the public will be of primary focus and concern.

Contributing to this change in locus of control is an increasing disillusionment and disenchantment with traditional health professionals, especially physicians. According to Alberta Health (1993, p. 7), "Albertans increasingly realize there is more to good health than health care services." As Lynn M. Cook, Vice President (Corporate Development) at the University of Alberta Hospital, observes, "There is no doubt in my mind that total quality management is the approach to take because of the focus on the customer. By always recycling back to find out what is important to the customer and delivering that in an excellent way, we are going to be able to improve service and sustain the health care system. The system will only be delivering those things that the customers find of value. It is happening already. The strength of the professions is being eroded because the public no longer sees it as sacrosanct to challenge the health care providers" (dialogue with the executive team, December 6, 1993).

As the professionals are being challenged, so are the unions. In Worster's (1993, p. 12) assessment, unions must revisit and revitalize their roles: "Having addressed the wrongs of the last century, [unions] must resort to portraying the worker as the victim and management as the enemy in order to keep themselves in business. . . . Unionism, like the federal bureaucracy, is one of the last bastions of socialism. In collective bargaining, all wages are averaged out, with the least productive worker being paid the same as the most productive. Hard work and personal ambition are discouraged in favor of dependence on the union for 'protection.'"

As the implications of rigid collective agreements play themselves out in an era of cutbacks and constraint, the public and health care workers are coming to the conclusion that the old paradigm of adversarial confrontation between unions and employing organizations is no longer effective. Unions are demonstrating interest in forging new relationships with the system through such processes as mutual gains bargaining.

Members of the public are not exempt from the need to revisit their expectations of the health care system. There is a need for "society" to redefine realistic expectations related to the costs and benefits of interventions, describe basic health services, and encourage and promote personal responsibility for maintenance of healthy lifestyles. "Society" must become involved with health professionals in assessing the ethical implications of particular actions and interventions. As Etzioni (1993) postulates, "Strong rights presume strong responsibilities." Inasmuch as comprehensive health care is viewed as a right of citizenship, the responsibility to make wise and prudent use of the resource is an obligation. Just as there are expectations of the health care professionals to generate knowledge about outcomes and quality of care, at the same time it is the responsibility of every member of society to ensure wise, ethical, and prudent use of health care resources.

Social expectations surrounding remuneration of health care professionals will also be on the agenda. The fee-for-service payment scheme is viewed as being at odds with health goals. It is a system that promotes volume in an era when cost constraint and quality point to different values.

System Financing

The fifth pillar of health care reform pertains to the financing of the system of care delivery. Gaylin (1993) suggests four principal causes of soaring health costs, as presented earlier in this chapter: (1) increasing morbidity rates, (2) the expanding concept of health, (3) the seduction of technology, and (4) the perception that limits do not exist.

Southerst (1993, p. 1) presents another point of view: "Health-care costs in Canada are running out of control for a simple reason:

our fee-for-service system, doctors, labs and hospitals perform services and governments pay for them. The more providers do, the more they get paid. It's a blueprint for aggressive medicine, replete with marginally useful tests, surgery, and hospital care." Both perspectives must be addressed.

The existential questions associated with Gaylin's four principal causes of overspending will take society a long time to address and will be complex. However, the fiscal challenges will force the setting of priorities that remained unestablished throughout times of plenty. As issues of national and provincial debt are addressed in Canada, financial resources available for health care are diminishing. It is planned that, over a three-year period, government spending on health care will be reduced by 17.6 percent, or $734 million (Government of Alberta, 1994).

Not only will the fiscal situation force consideration of Gaylin's existential issues, the basic principles of the Canadian health care system will be revisited. Definition of basic health will be required, user fees will be considered, and more dependence on charitable donations and revenue generation will challenge the public funding tenet of the system as we know it.

In addressing the fee-for-service characteristics associated with the provision of services, changes are already under consideration. An alternate payment plan for physicians is a topic that arises at every forum addressing health care reform. As laboratory, radiology and imaging, and "medi center" services undergo scrutiny, the need to finance such services through very different methods becomes increasingly evident. The government has stated that, in the near future, all funding for health-related services will be channeled through regional boards. They, in turn, will have the authority to allocate the funds in a manner that most appropriately meets the needs of the communities they serve.

As the various possibilities for health care reform become clearer to leaders and change agents currently associated with organizations delivering some facet of the service to consumers, the tasks ahead appear formidable. Many are bewildered in terms of knowing how to approach the future or respond to the changes. Others view total quality management as equipping organizations and individuals with the tools they need to proceed with confidence and creativity.

Confronting the Challenges: Total Quality Management

Total quality management, as it has been defined and presented in this book and implemented at the University of Alberta Hospital, assumes a very broad perspective on the concept. Encompassing continuous improvement and reengineering, total quality management, as viewed through the three domains of the Organization Capability Development Framework, provides the philosophy and principles through which to address the challenges of the past that will continue to be encountered, the activities of the present, and the health care and social reform challenges of the future.

The need for fundamental change is clear. Total quality management provides principles that assist in addressing the challenges that are currently being and will continue to be faced in health care: How do we empower our staff in decision making? How do we promote the effective relationships necessary for forwarding action? How do we align our systems; focus on customer satisfaction; measure the outcomes of our interventions; collaborate effectively with our partners? In all of this, what about accountability and teamwork? How do we equip organizations to move forward with a commitment to ongoing learning? All of these questions must be addressed if we are to successfully respond to the formidable challenges of the future.

As Davidson observes, total quality management, in its broadest definition, is the tool that can transform health care. "But you need to look at it in a bigger framework, and our Organization Capability Development Framework consisting of context, infrastructure, and member capability is proving to be an excellent transformational model" (dialogue with the executive team, December 6, 1993). As Taylor suggests, "quality can be the vehicle to transform health care, as long as you make it *the* vehicle to transform health care. If you treat it as an "add on" or as an initiative among many, it will not be successful. It works at the University of Alberta Hospital because we have made it our major effort" (dialogue with the executive team, December 6, 1993). The challenge now is system reform.

Cook makes the following observation: "The power of the quality approach to transform health care is the focus on the customer. I think the customers will transform the system and we have seen a lot of evidence of that: disenchantment with physicians, people looking for alternate types of health care delivery—acupuncture and holistic medicine, for example. There is no doubt in my mind that the quality approach is the one to take because of this focus on the customer—by always recycling back to find out what is important to the customer and delivering it in an excellent way" (dialogue with the executive team, December 6, 1993).

Kofman and Senge (1993) present a compelling perspective related to the commitment of those participating in the organization. As with Gaylin (1993) and McKnight (1994), they anticipate that the success of organizations in transformation and learning is contingent upon the ability to deal with fundamental cultural dysfunction:

> Building learning organizations, we are discovering, requires basic shifts in how we think and interact. The changes go beyond individual corporate cultures, or even the culture of Western management; they penetrate to the bedrock assumptions and habits of our culture as a whole. We are also discovering that moving forward is an exercise in personal commitment and community building. As Dr. W. Edwards Deming says, nothing happens without "personal transformation."

As the challenges, constraints, and successes associated with organizational transformation have become increasingly understood by the executive team within the hospital, the fundamental importance of personal transformation in forwarding organizational change has become evident. Unless we can deal effectively with the three areas of cultural dysfunction—fragmentation, competition, and reactiveness—as described by Kofman and Senge (1993), the ability to successfully transform organizations will be significantly compromised. This is a challenge for the entire system of health care and, more broadly, for society as a whole.

The executive team at the University of Alberta Hospital is unified in its commitment that total quality management, as described here, is sufficient to the challenges that lie ahead. However, effecting the fundamental cultural change advocated by Kofman and Senge (1993) is a formidable task, one that cannot be taken on in isolation.

Is total quality management sufficient to enable us to confront the challenge? The principles of total quality management provide a powerful approach to promote the systemic, cultural, and societal change advocated by many. We have seen evidence and demonstrated results to indicate that change is beginning. However, the key to fundamental transformation is the commitment to personal transformation of each individual occupying a role in the organization, the health care system, and indeed society as a whole.

As the challenges of the past and present have been reviewed and as the specific aspects of health care reform have been anticipated, the associated process has brought the authors of this book to an even deeper commitment to the total quality management philosophy and approach as the one viable alternative to meet the demands and challenges anticipated in the future. Through total quality management, we expect to create the future through positive, creative, and proactive actions rather than allow the wonderful health care system that Canadians have come to value and appreciate to be destroyed.

References

Alberta Health. *Health Goals for Alberta: A Progress Report.* Edmonton: Government of Alberta, 1993.

Berwick, D. "Improving Community Health Status." *Quality Connection,* 1993, *2*(4), 2–3.

Blackburn, R. S., and Ridky, J. "Changing Managerial Paradigms." In J. Ridky and G. F. Sheldon (eds.), *Managing in Academics: A Health Center Model.* St. Louis, Mo.: Quality Medical Publishing, 1993.

Blumenthal, D., and Meyer, G. S. "The Future of the Academic Medical Center Under Health Care Reform." *New England Journal of Medicine,* 1993, *329*(24), 1812–1814.

Byrne, J. A. "The Horizontal Corporation: It's About Managing Across, Not Up and Down." *Business Week,* December 20, 1993, pp. 76–81.

Etzioni, A. *The Spirit of Community.* New York: Simon and Schuster, 1993.

Gaylin, W. "Faulty Diagnosis: Why Clinton's Health-care Plan Won't Cure What Ails Us." *Harper's Magazine,* October 1993, pp. 57–64.

Government of Alberta. "Health Minister Outlines Three-Year Health Budget Targets." News release. Edmonton: Government of Alberta, January 18, 1994.

Hammer, M., and Champy, J. *Reengineering the Corporation: A Manifesto for Business Revolution.* New York: HarperCollins, 1993.

Kofman, F., and Senge, P. M. "Communities of Commitment: The Heart of Learning Organizations." In D. Bohl and F. Luthan (eds.), *Organizational Dynamics.* New York: American Management Association, 1993.

Joint Commission on Accreditation of Healthcare Organizations. *Accreditation Manual for Hospitals, Vol. 1: Standards.* Oakbrook Terrace, Ill.: Joint Commission on Accreditation, 1993, pp. 51–58.

McKnight, J. "Citizen, Government, and Community Reform." Lecture presented to health care workers at the Grey Nuns Hospital, Edmonton, Alberta, January 20, 1994.

Nash, D. B. "Bridging the Gap Between Theory and Practice: Exploring Clinical Practice Guidelines." *Joint Commission Journal on Quality Improvement,* 1993, *19*(9), 396–400.

Nelson, E. C. "Developing a Patient Measurement System for the Future: An Interview." *Joint Commission Journal on Quality Improvement,* 1993, *19*(9), 368–373.

O'Leary, D. S. "The Measurement Mandate: Report Card Day Is Coming." *The Joint Commission Journal on Quality Improvement,* 1993, *19*(11), 487–491.

Peters, T. *Thriving on Chaos.* New York: Knopf, 1987.

Scott, W. "Health Care Organizations in the 1980s: The Convergence of Public and Professional Control Systems." In J. W. Mayer and W. R. Scott (eds.), *Organizational Environments: Ritual and Rationality*. Newbury Park, Calif.: Sage, 1992.

Senge, P. M. "Transforming the Practice of Management." Paper presented at the Systems Thinking in Action Conference, Cambridge, Mass., November 14, 1991.

Southerst, J. "OK, Hillary, It's Our Turn." *Canadian Business*. December 1993, pp. 1–5.

Walzlawick, P., Weakland, J., and Fisch, R. *Change*. New York: W. W. Norton, 1974.

Worster, R. "Still Fighting Yesterday's Battle." *Newsweek*, Sept. 27, 1993, p. 12.

Index